PICTURE BOOK OF
SEWING

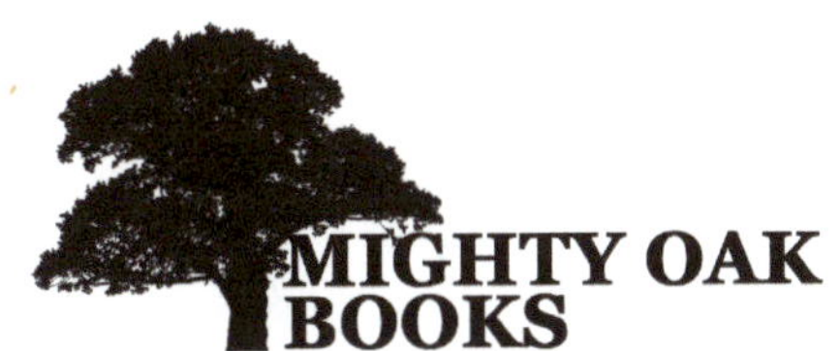

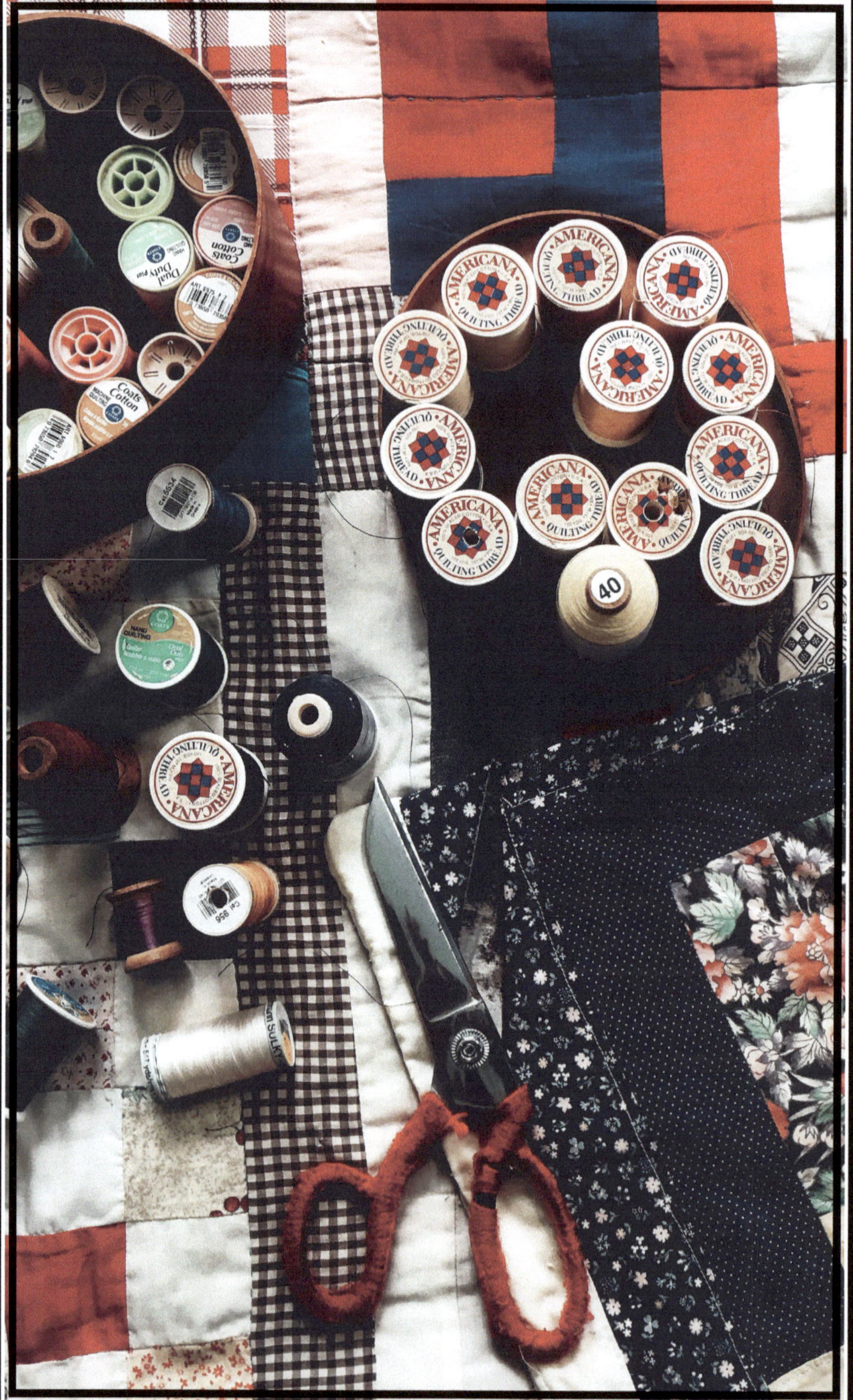

AMERICANA QUILTING THREAD
Coats Cotton
Dual Duty Plus
Coats Cotton
HAND QUILTING
40

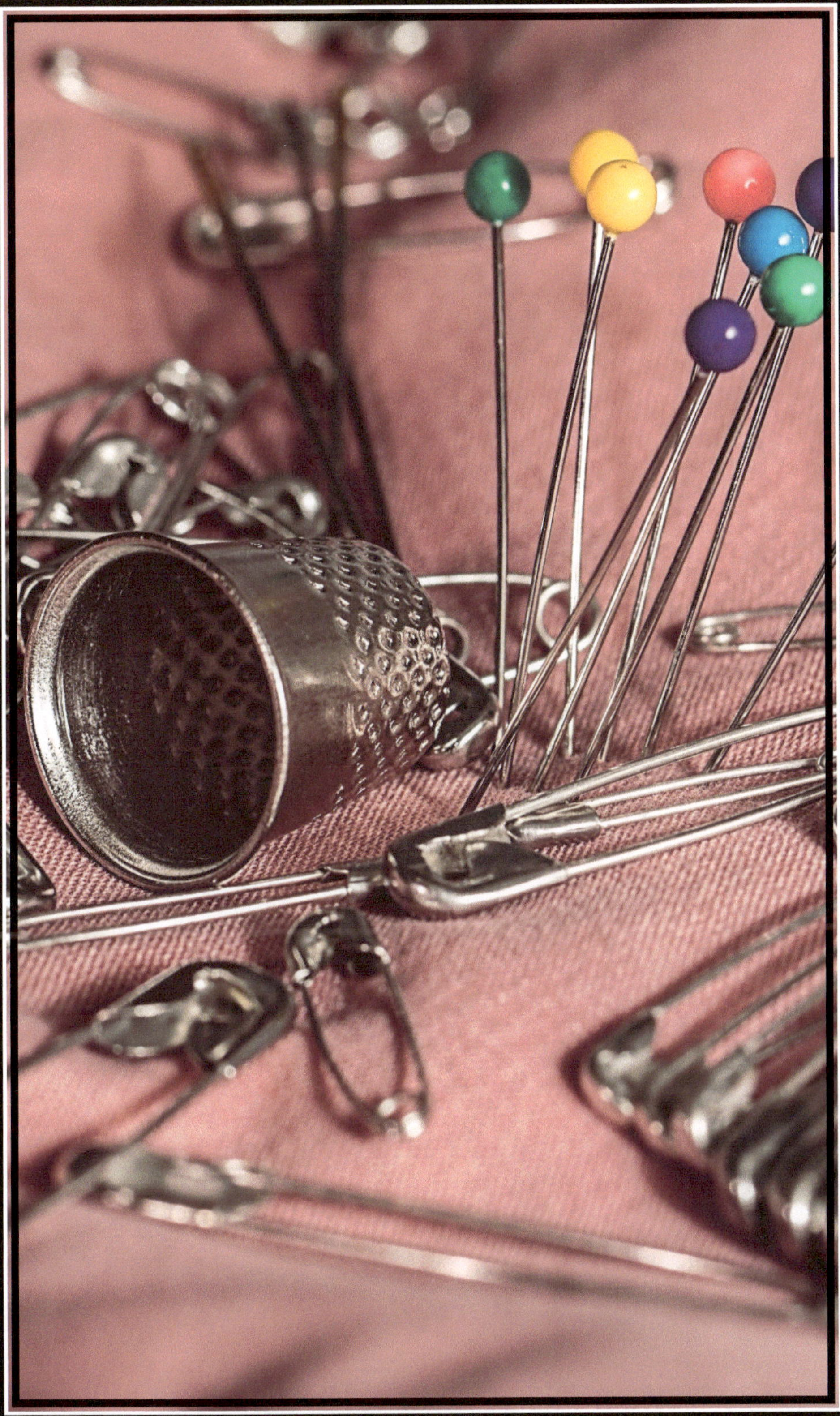

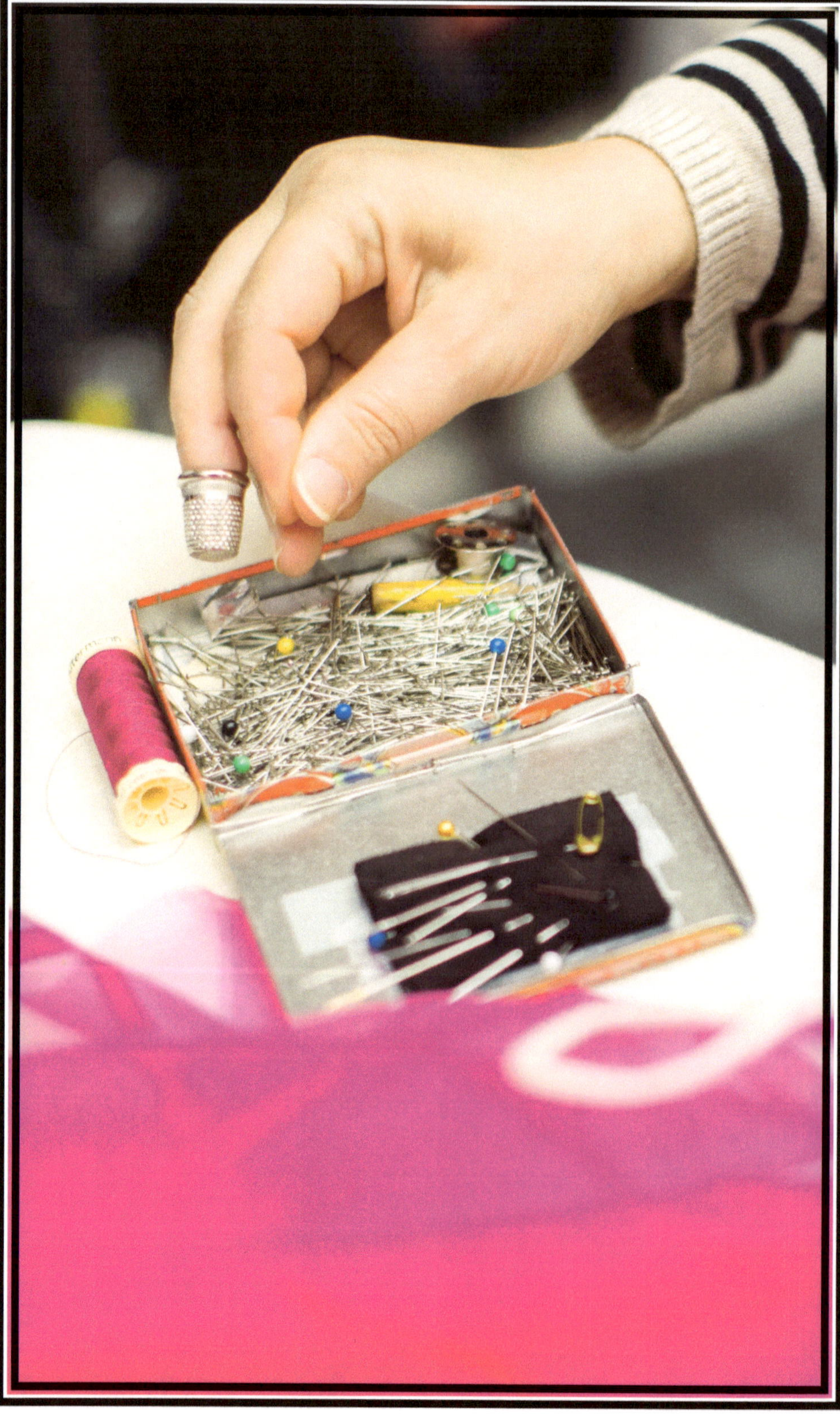

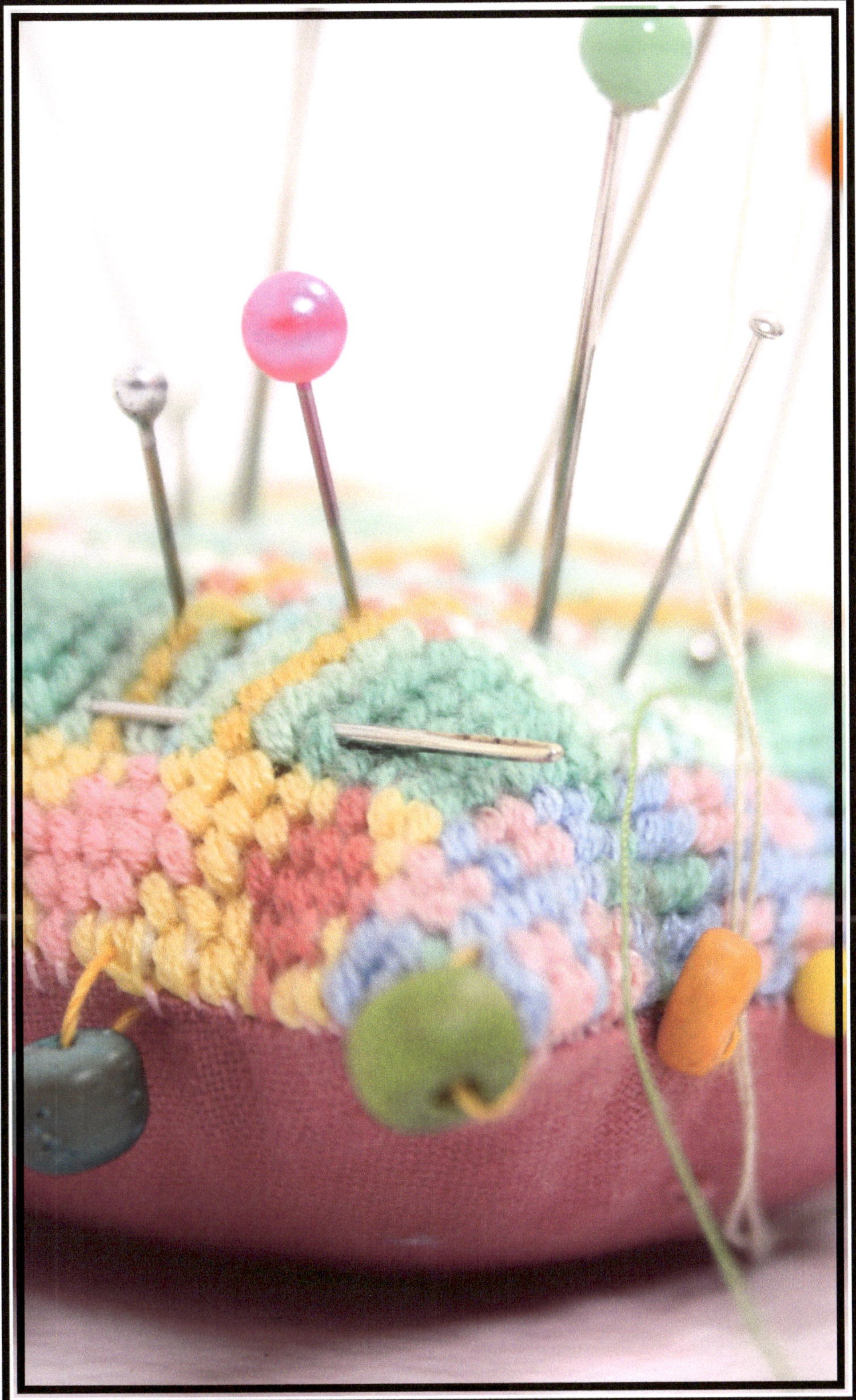

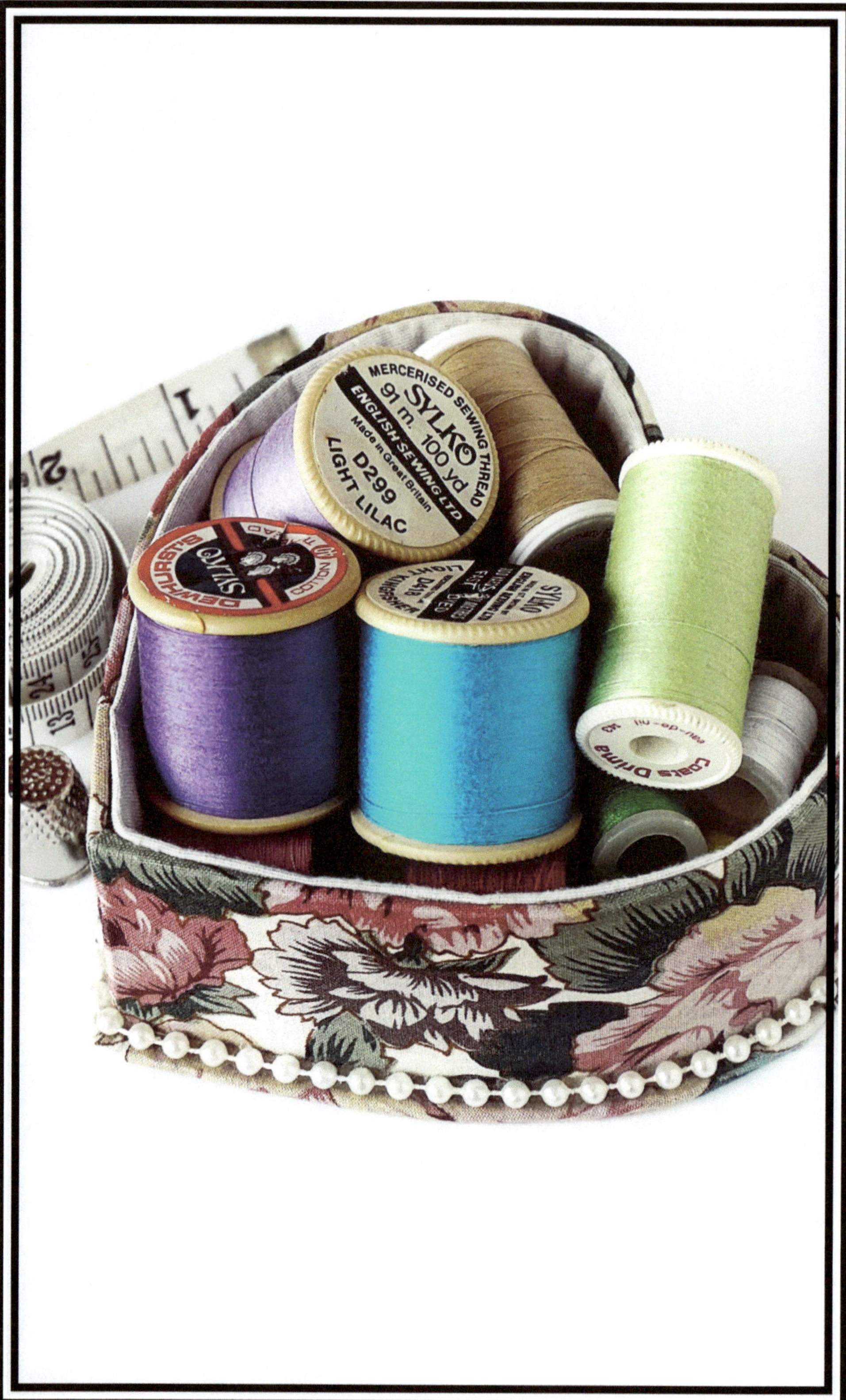

MERCERISED SEWING THREAD
SYLKO
91 m. 100 yd
Made in Great Britain
ENGLISH SEWING LTD
D299
LIGHT LILAC
DEWHURST'S SYLKO 40 COTTON
SYLKO
Coats Drima

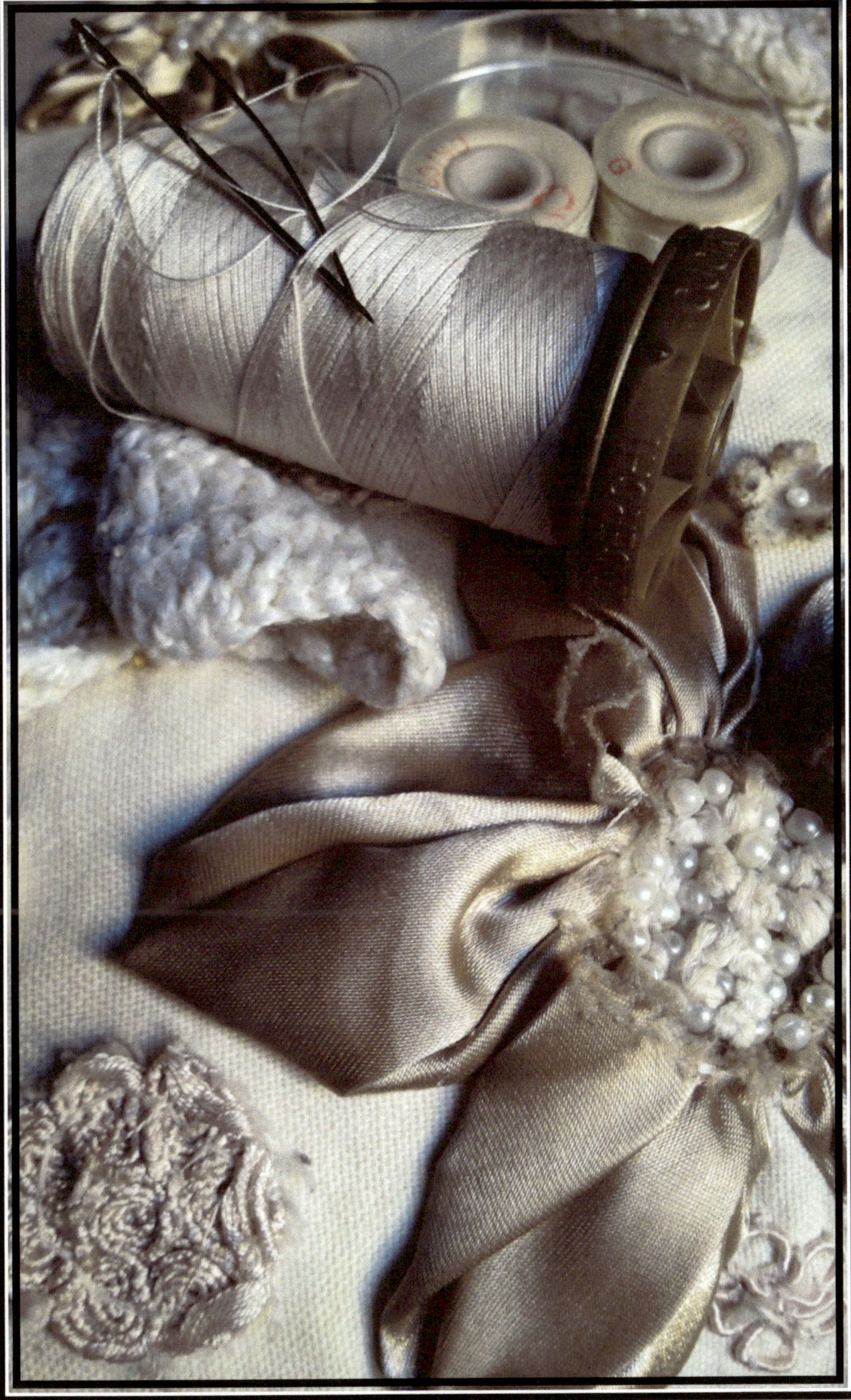

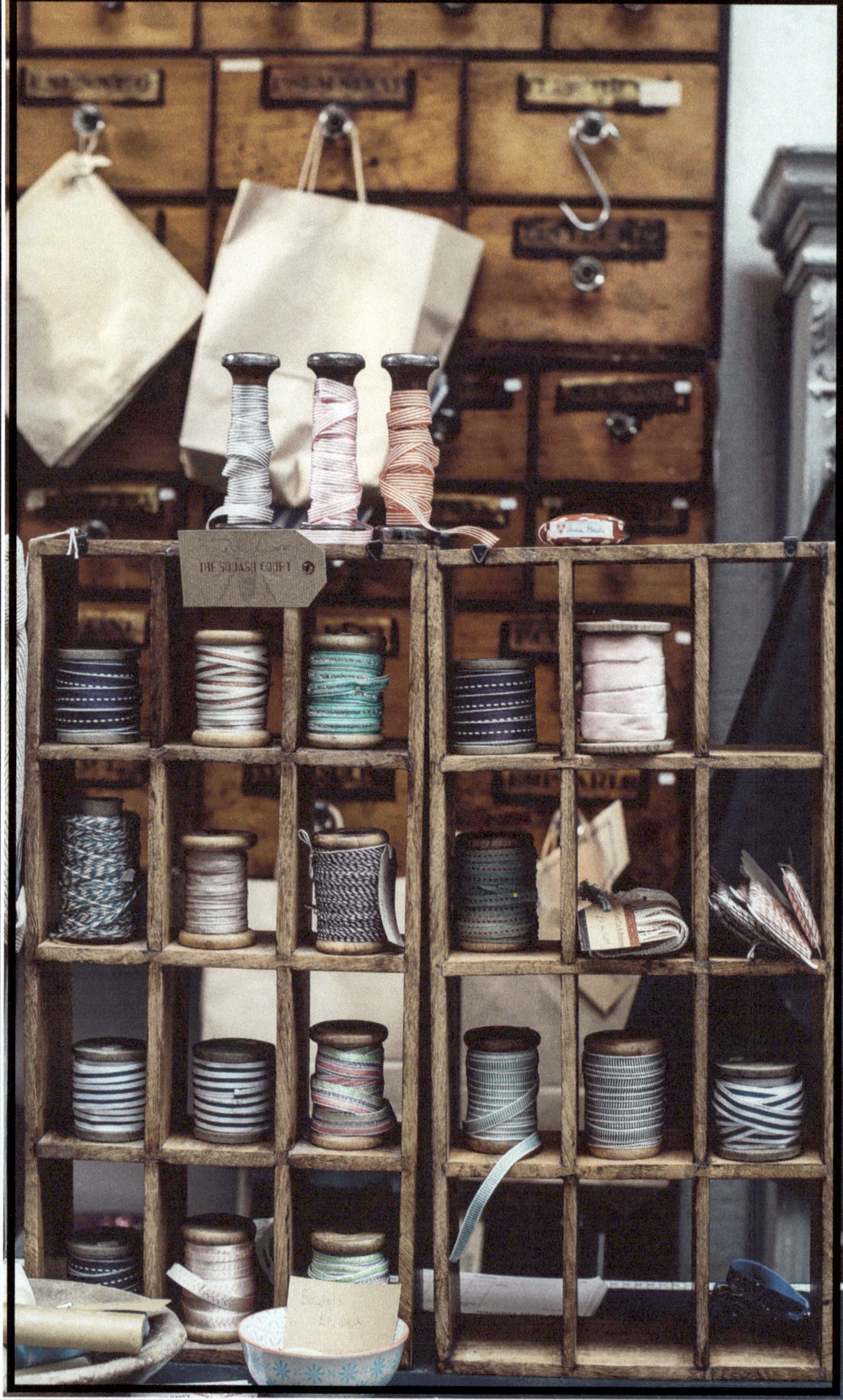
THE SQUASH COURT

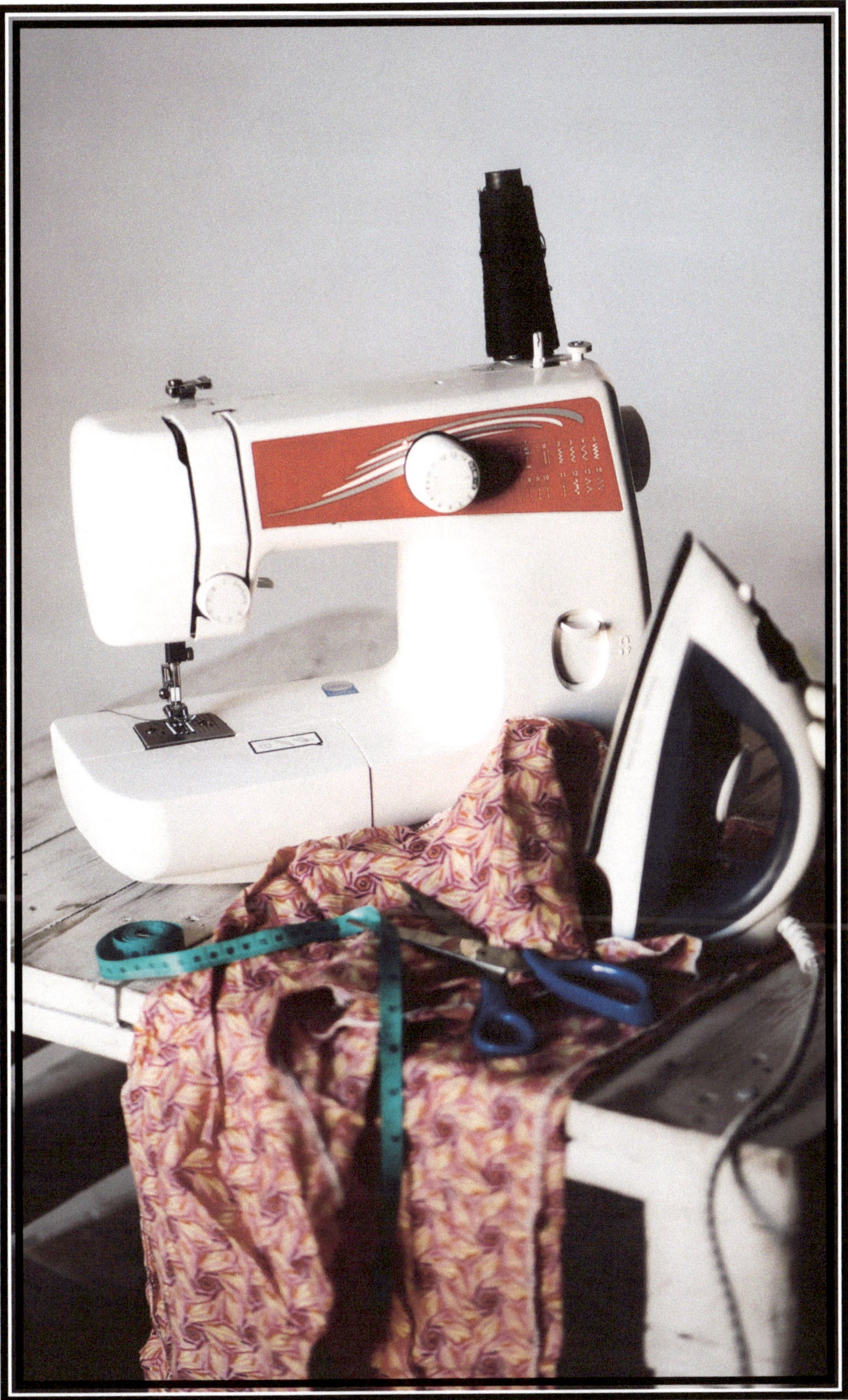

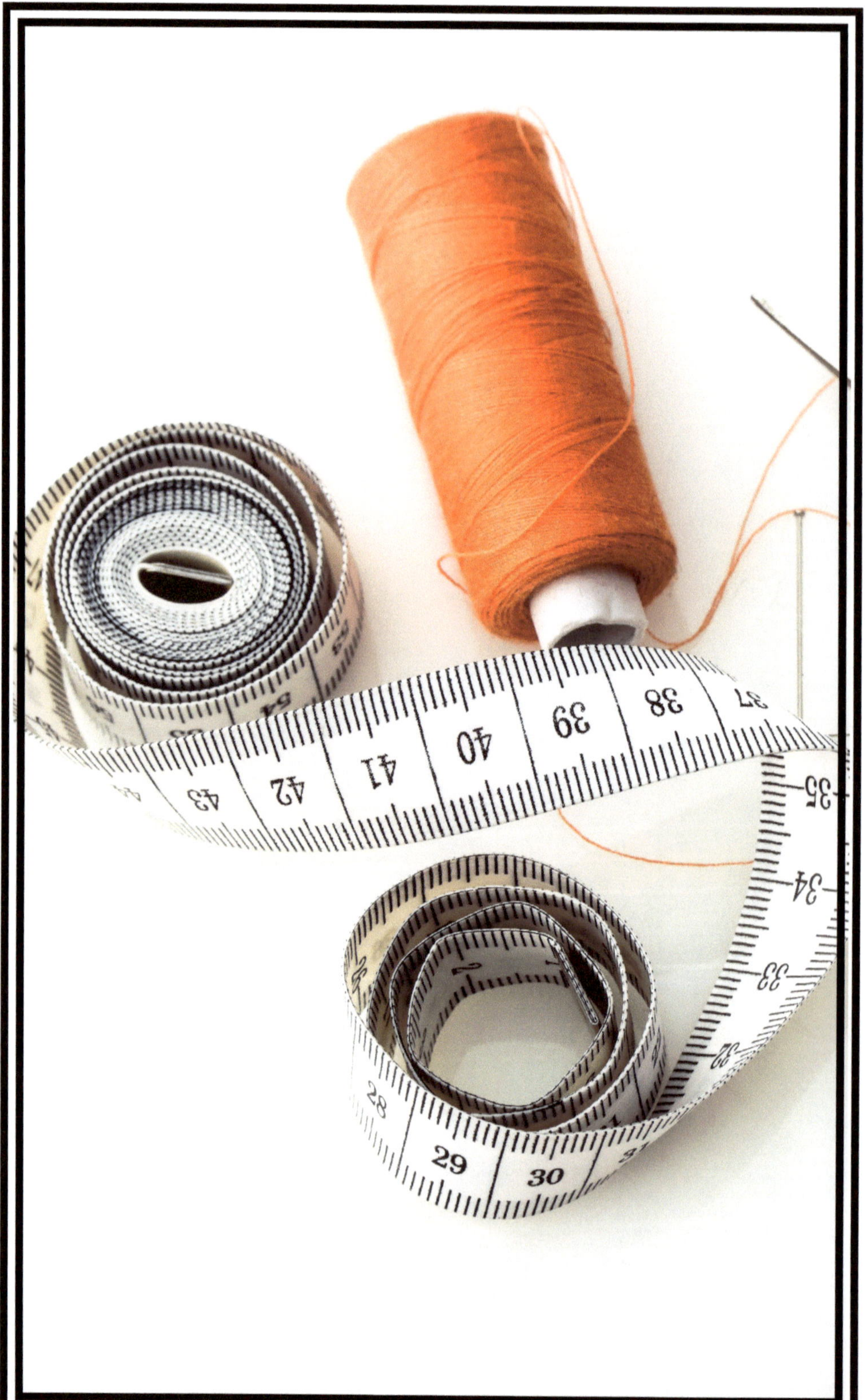

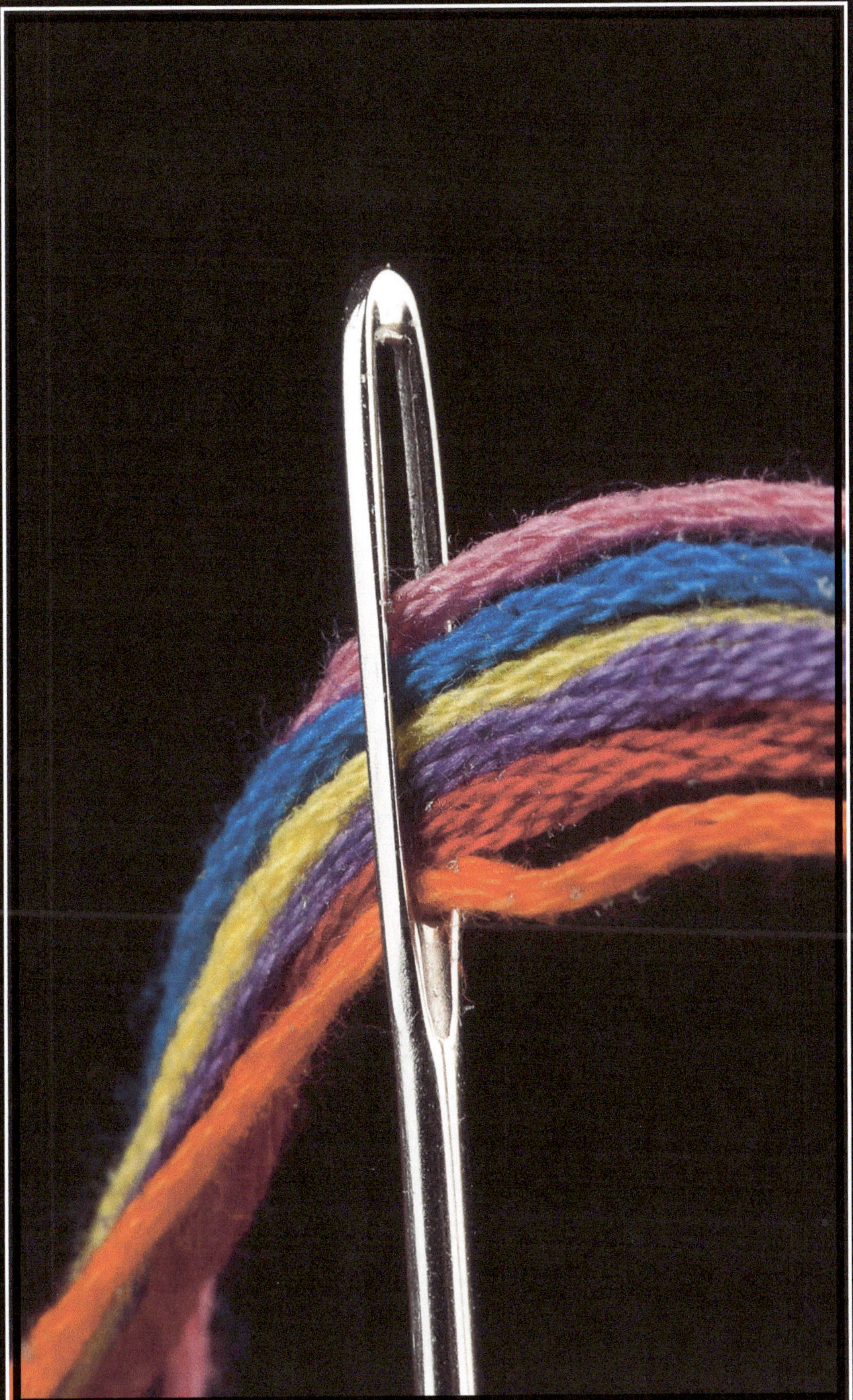

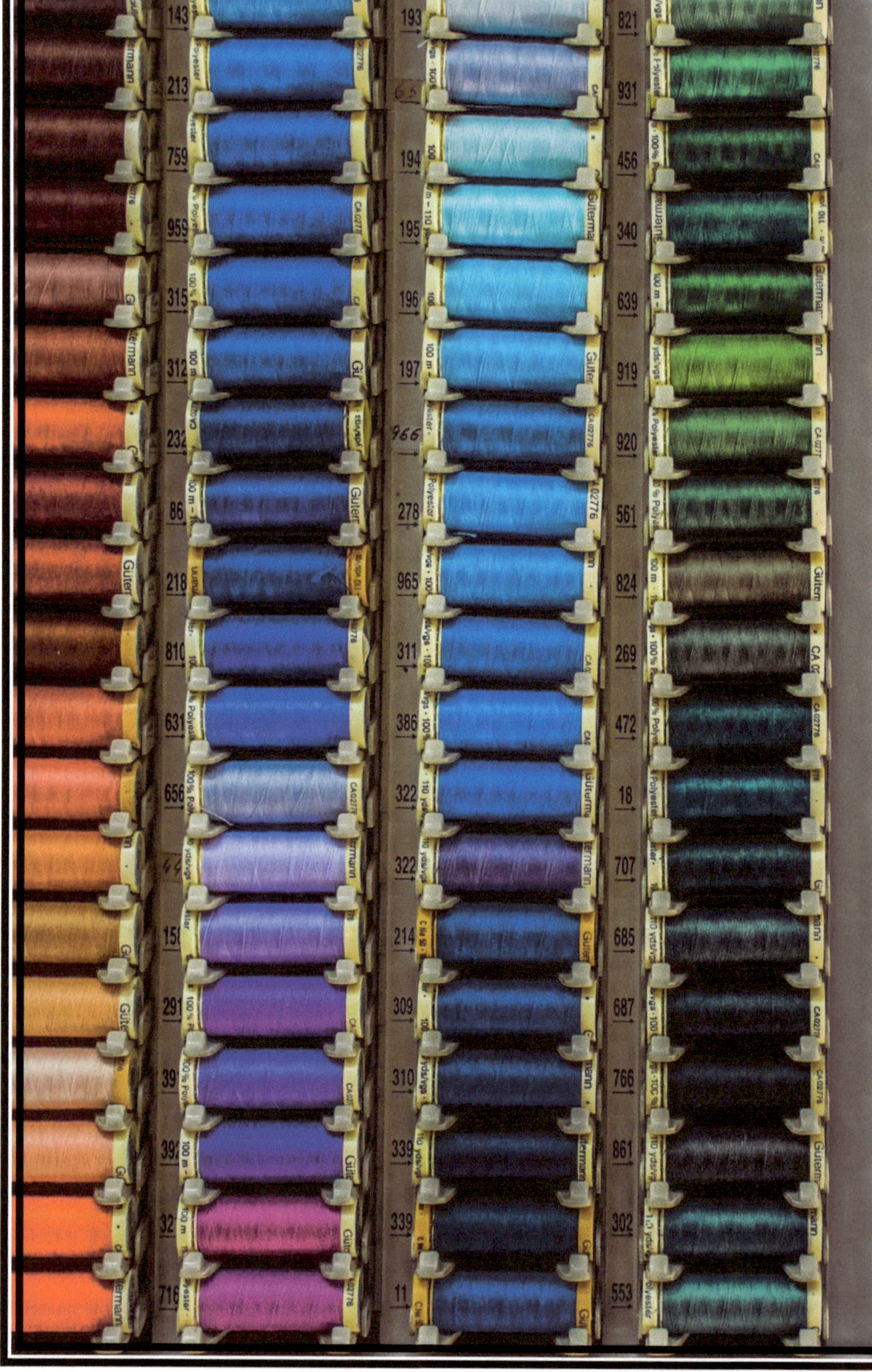

143
213
759
959
315
312
232
86
218
810
631
656
156
291
39
392
32
716
193
194
195
196
197
966
278
965
311
386
322
322
214
309
310
339
339
11
821
931
456
340
639
919
920
561
824
269
472
18
707
685
687
766
861
302
553

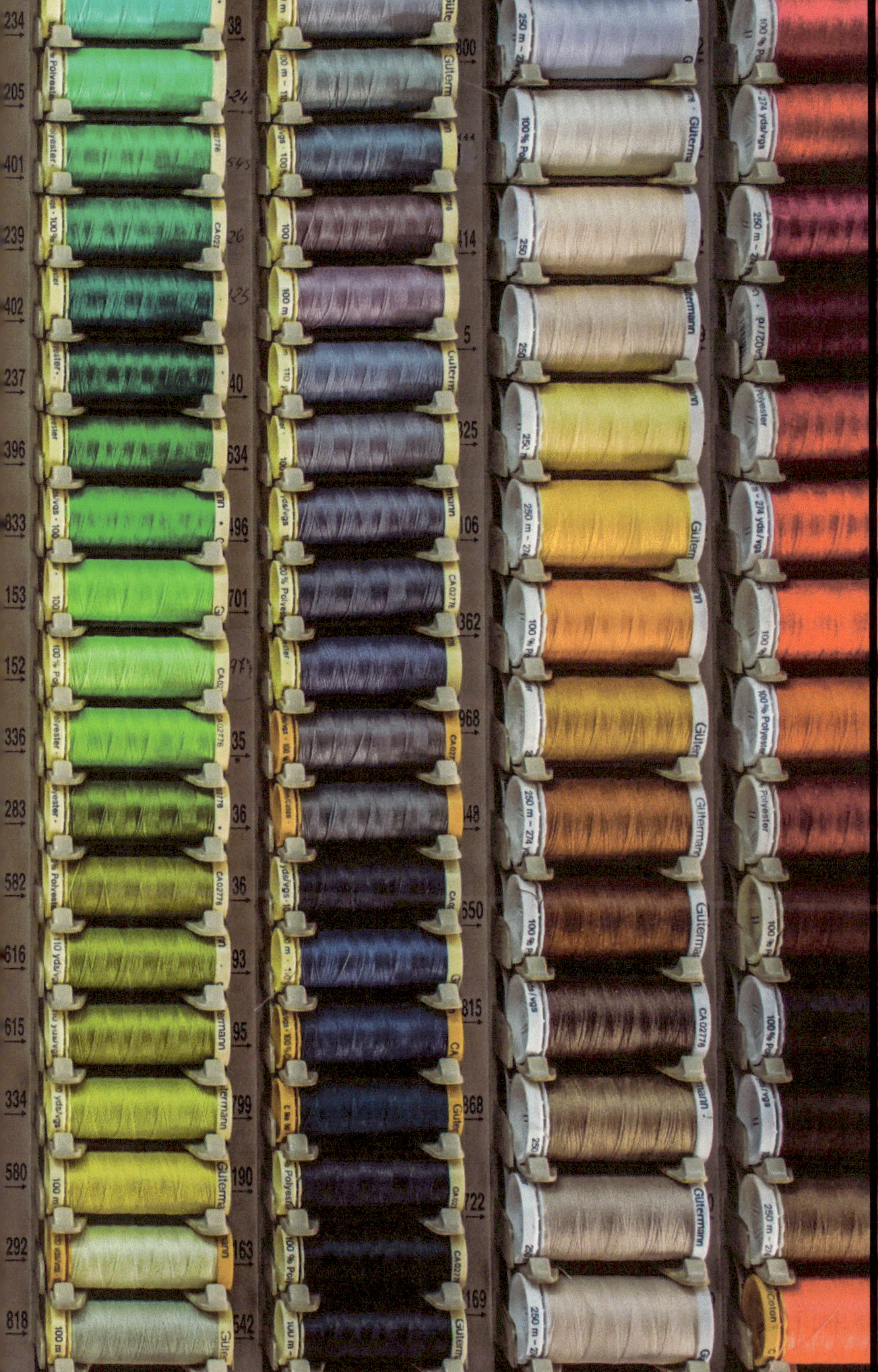

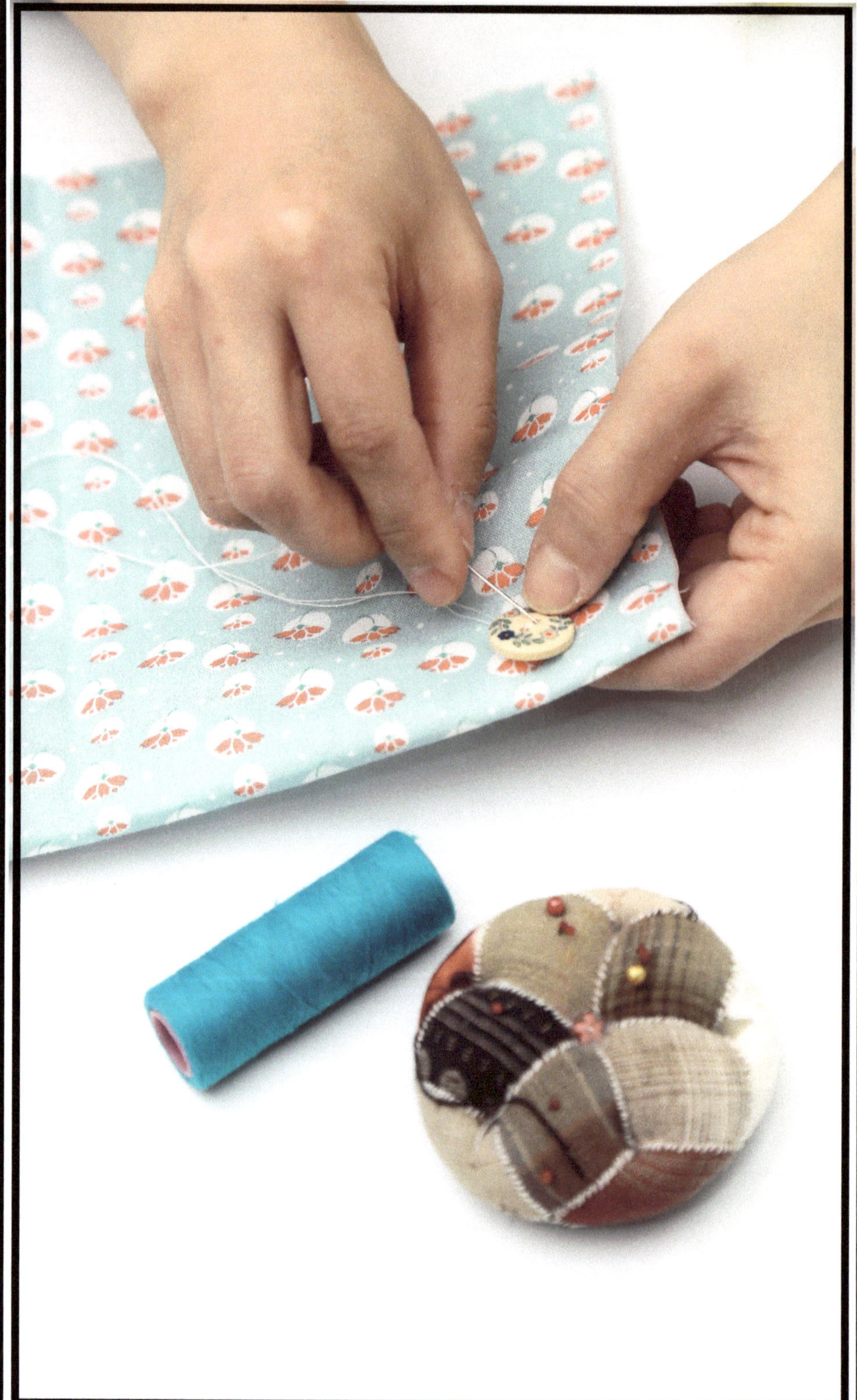

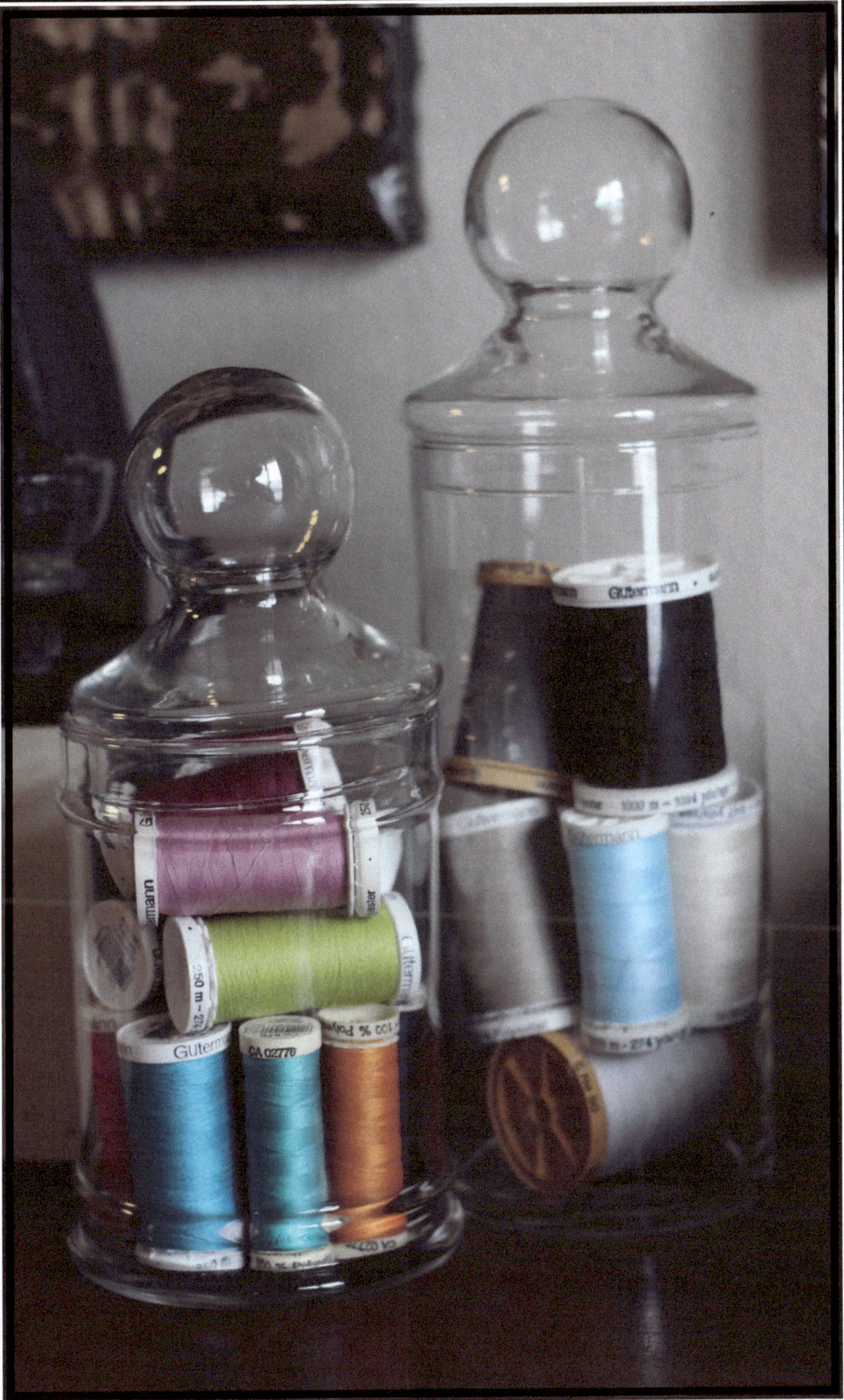

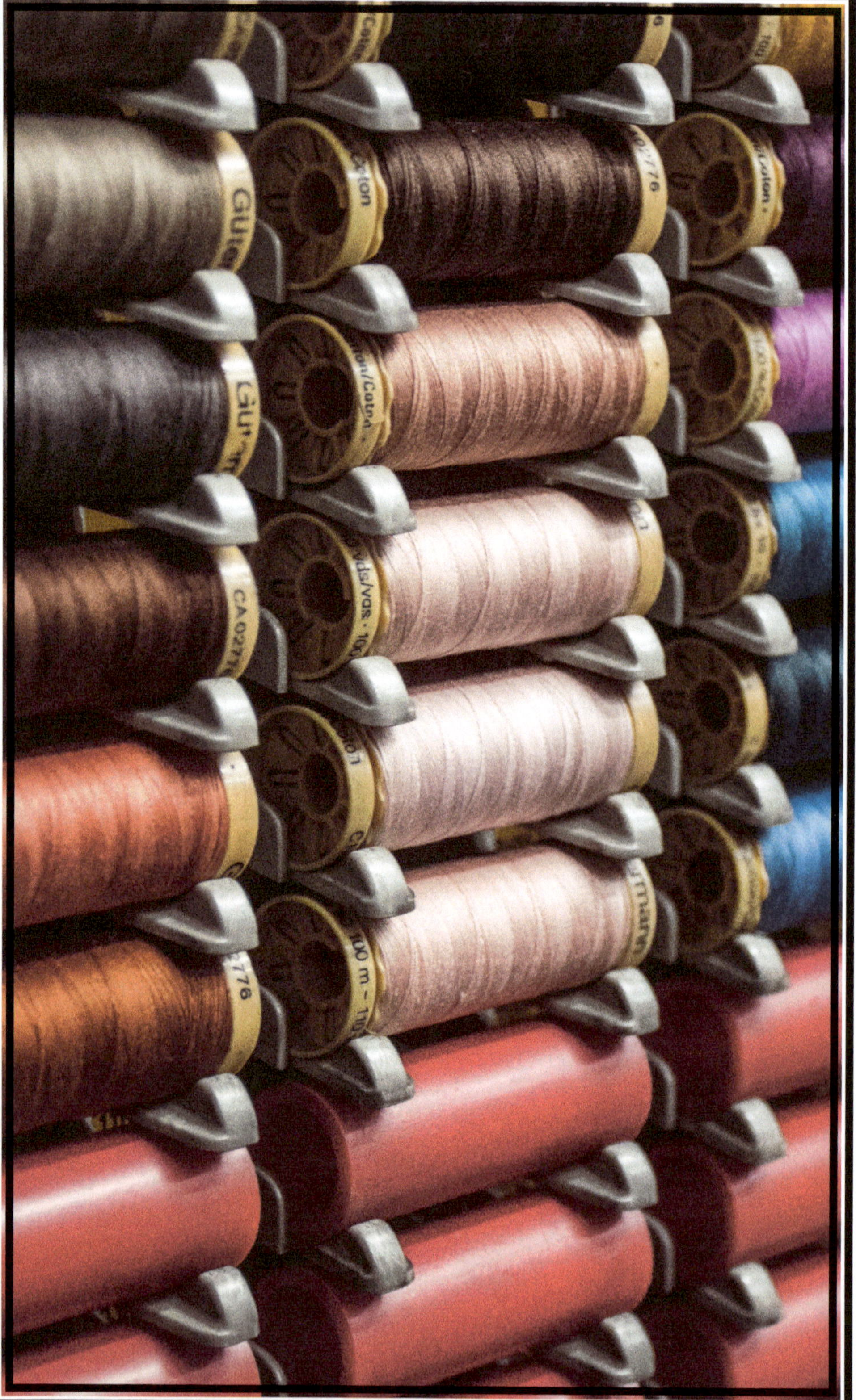

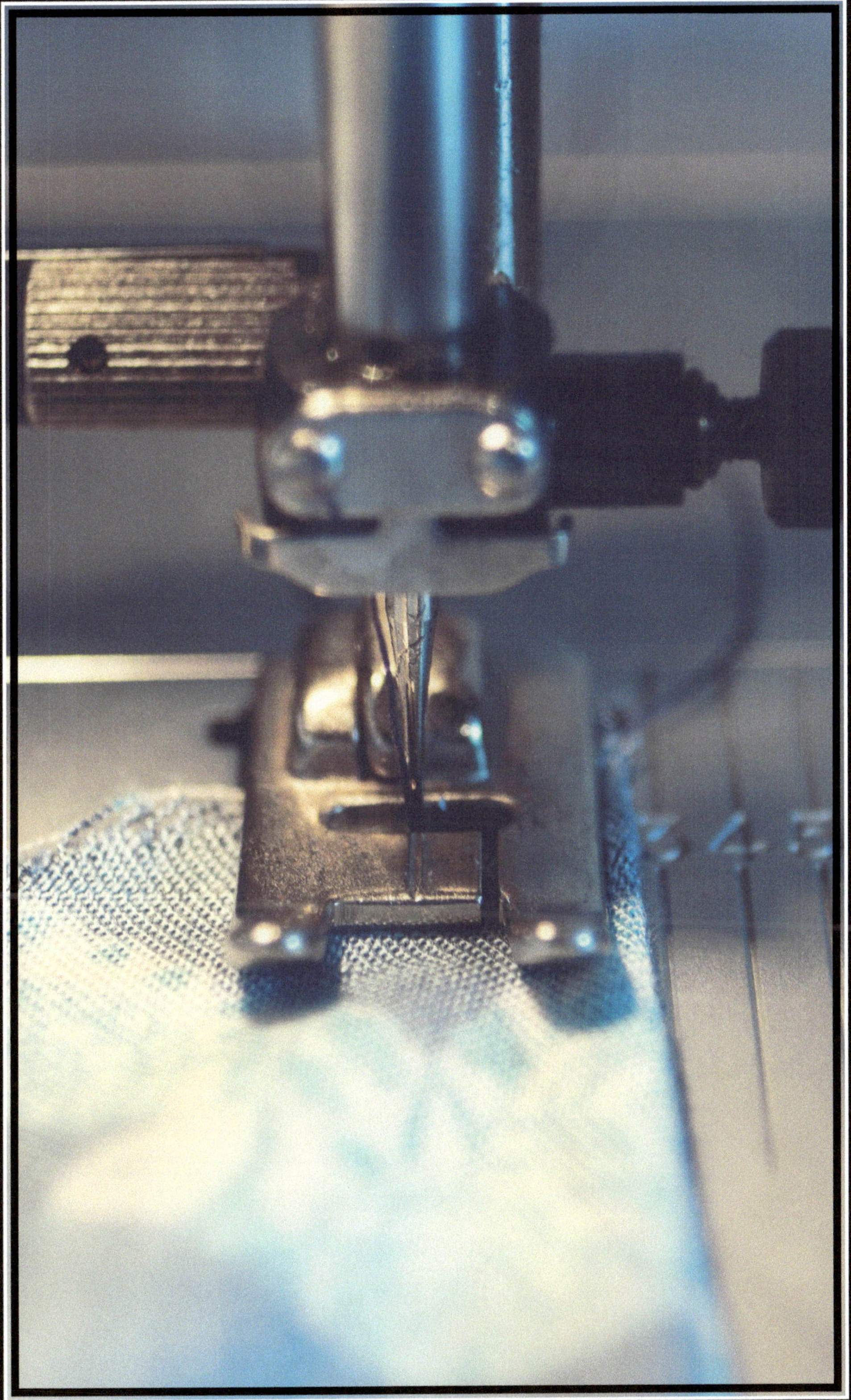

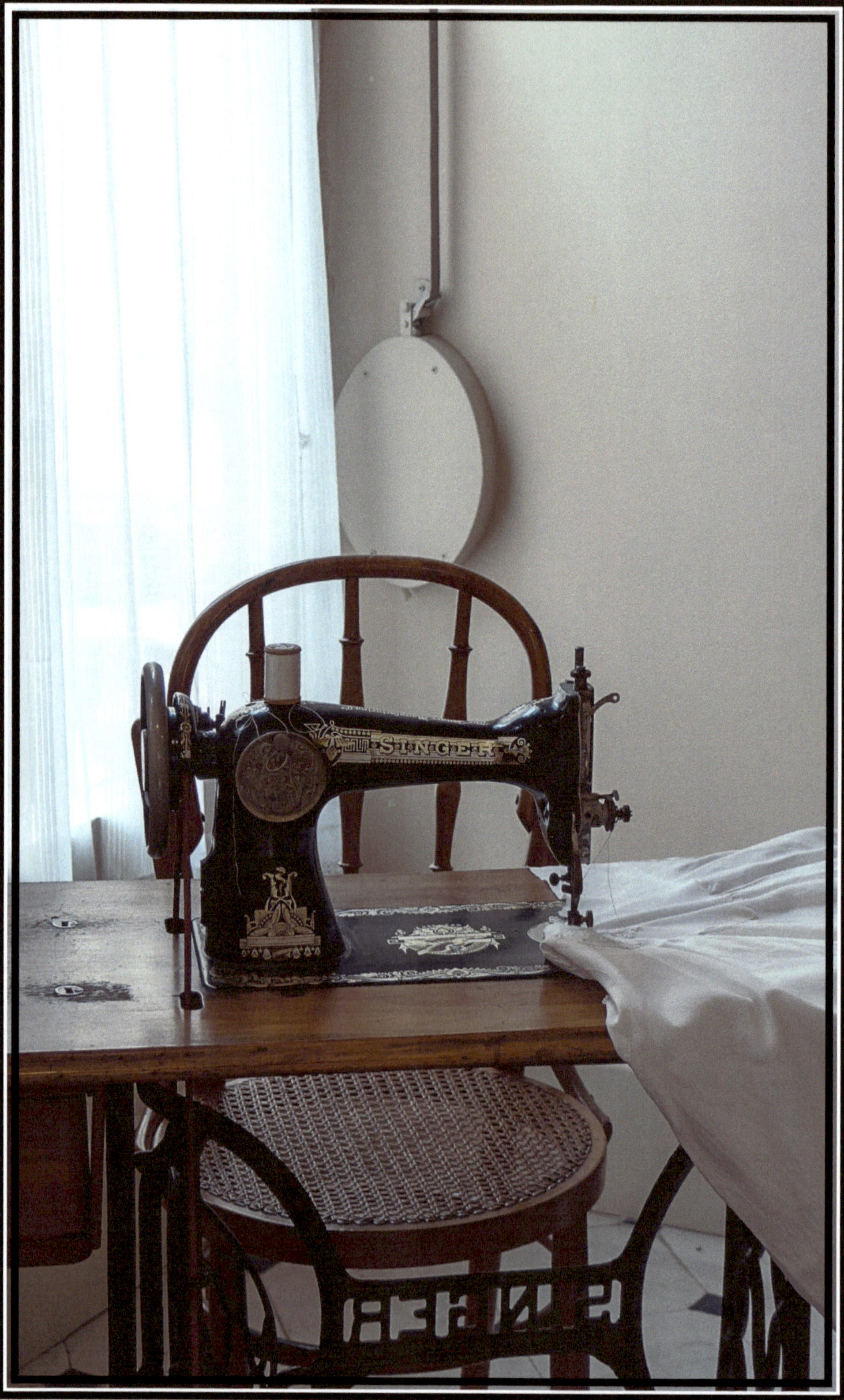

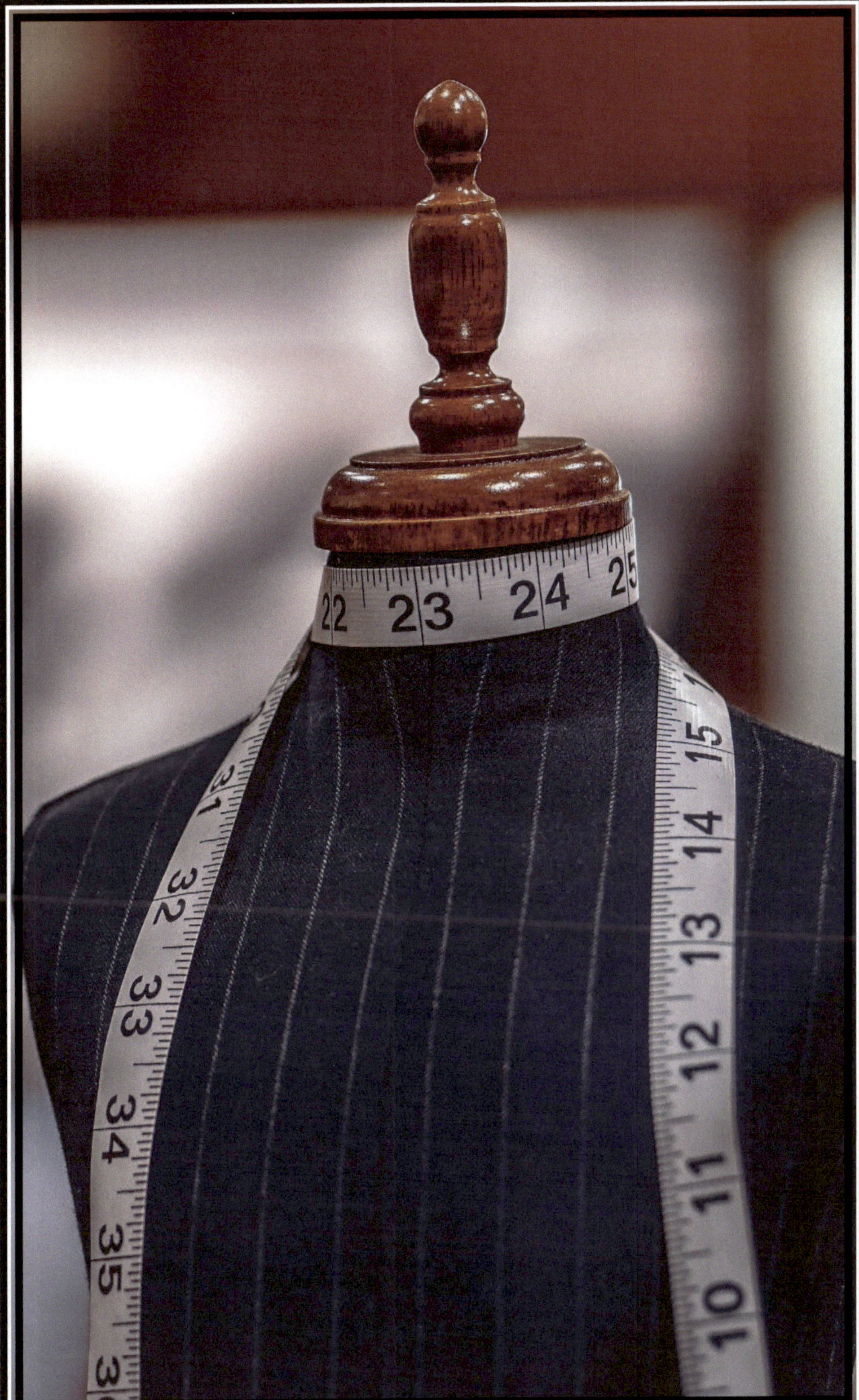

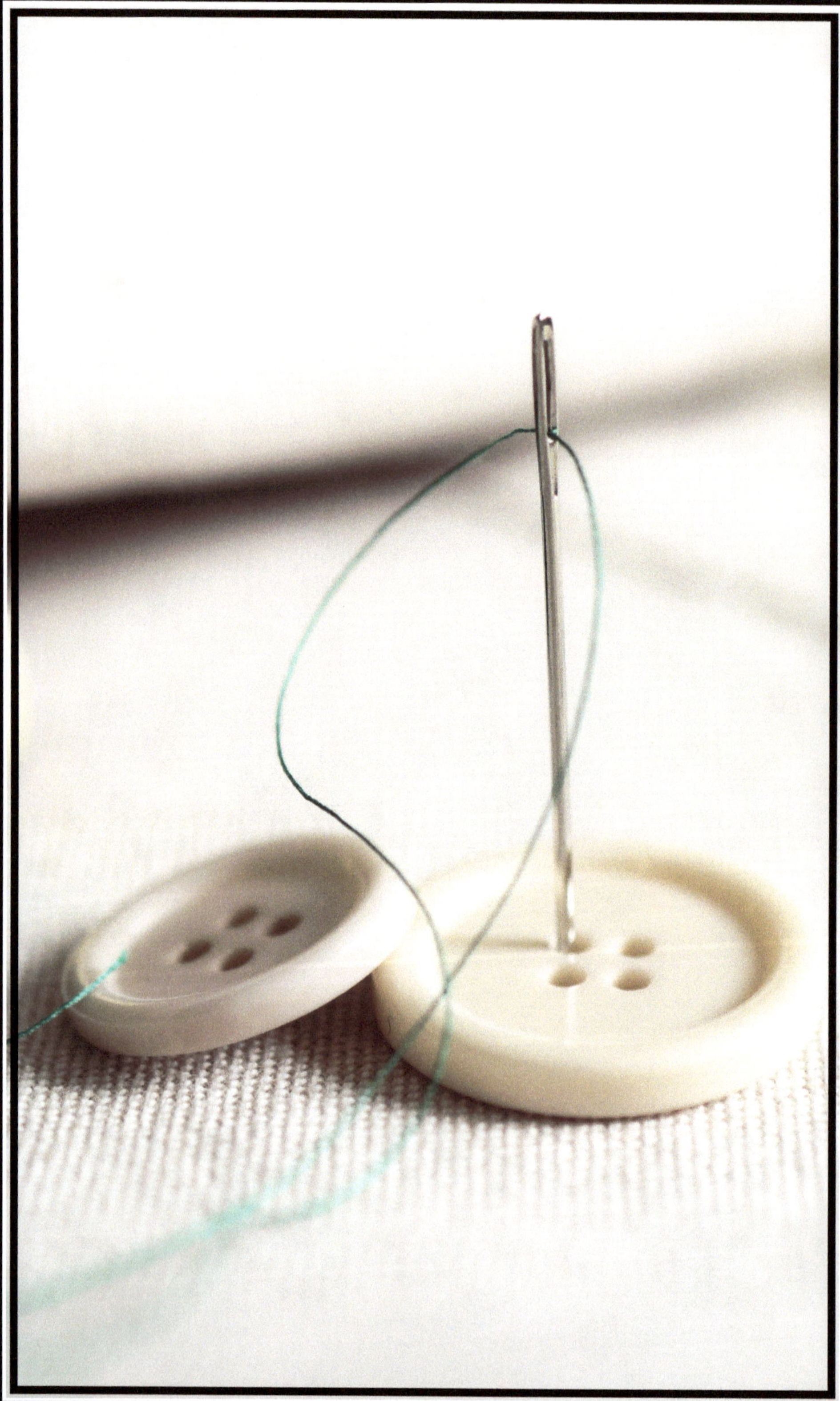

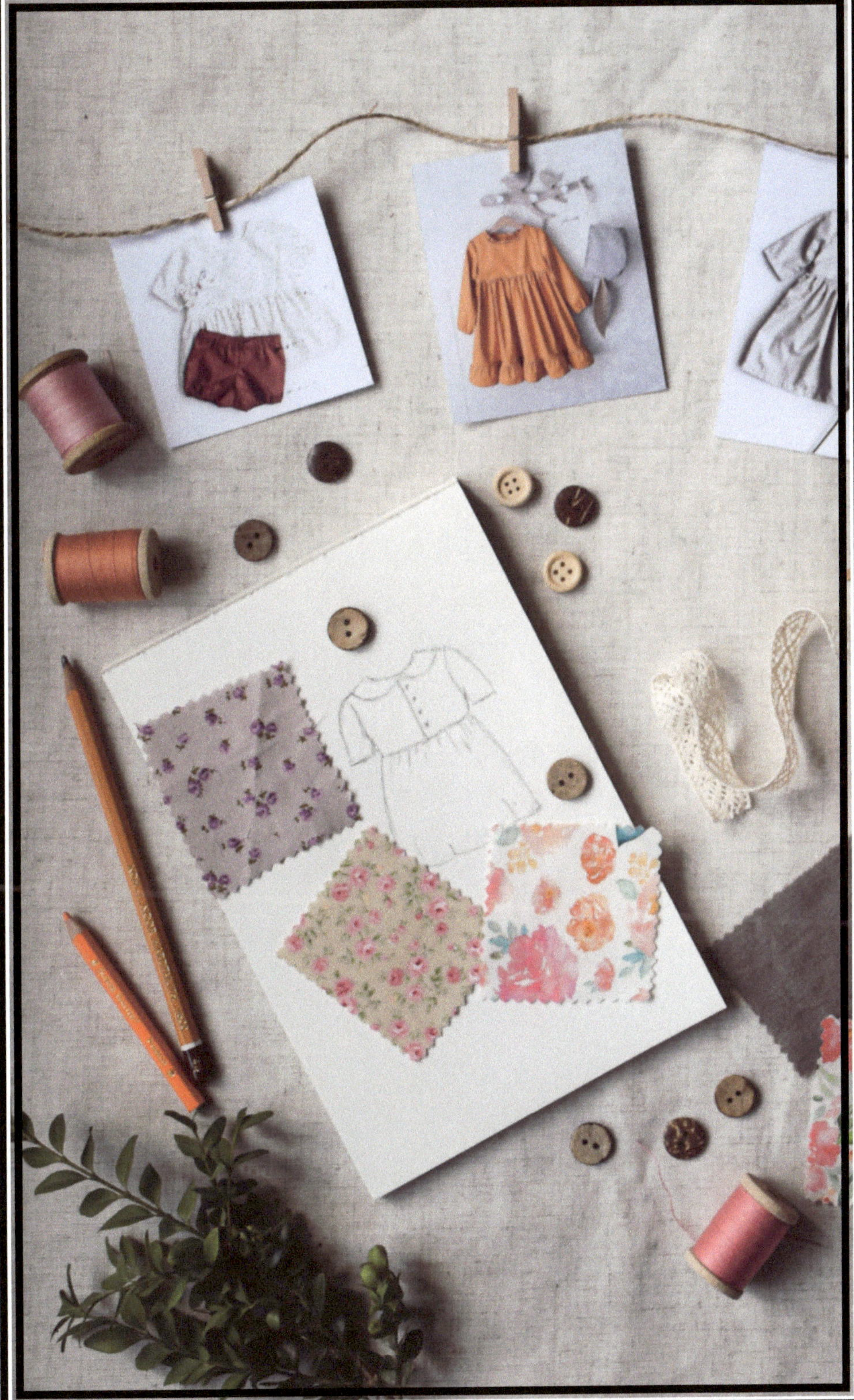

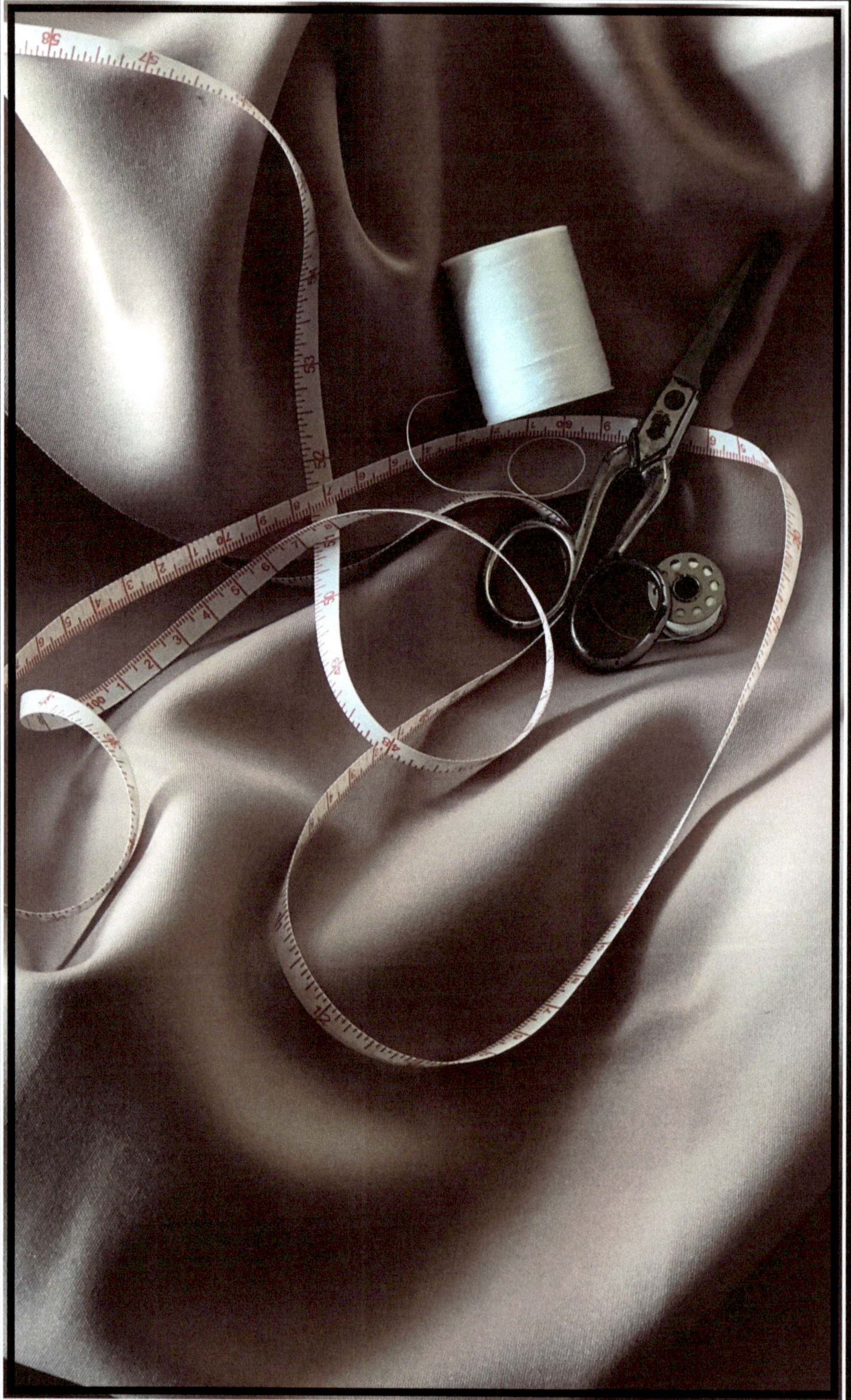

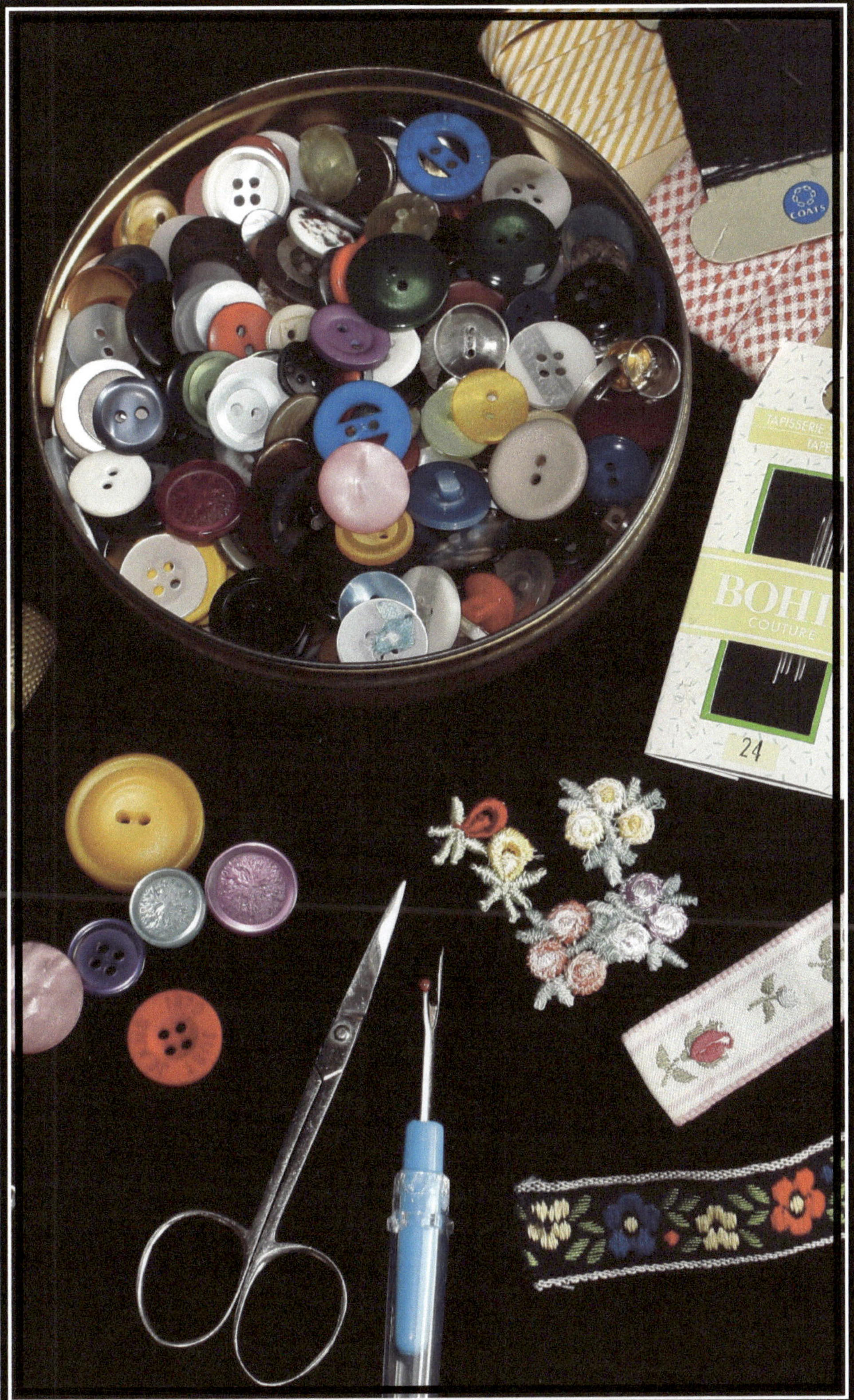
COATS
TAPISSERIE
TAPE
BOHI
COUTURE
24

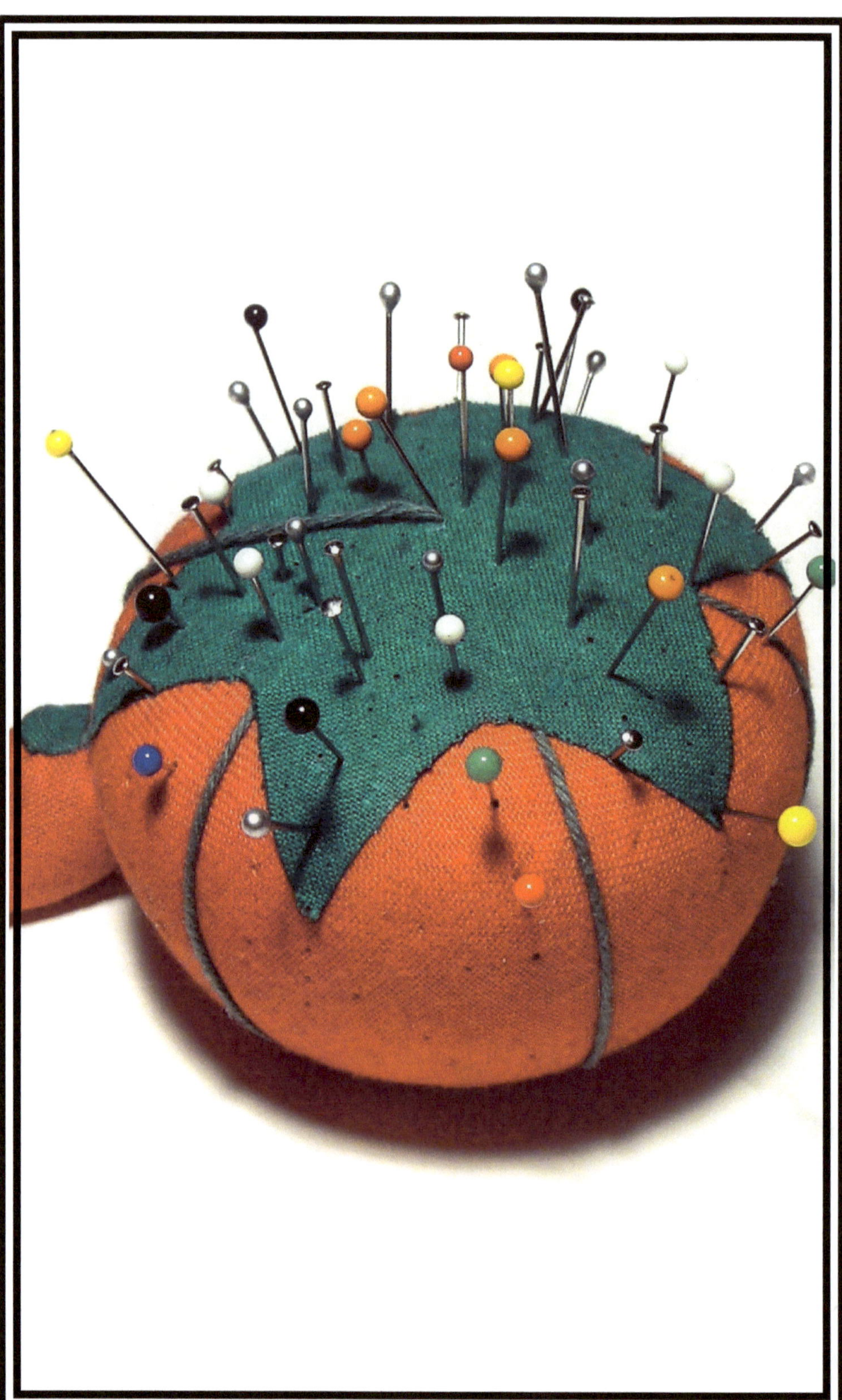

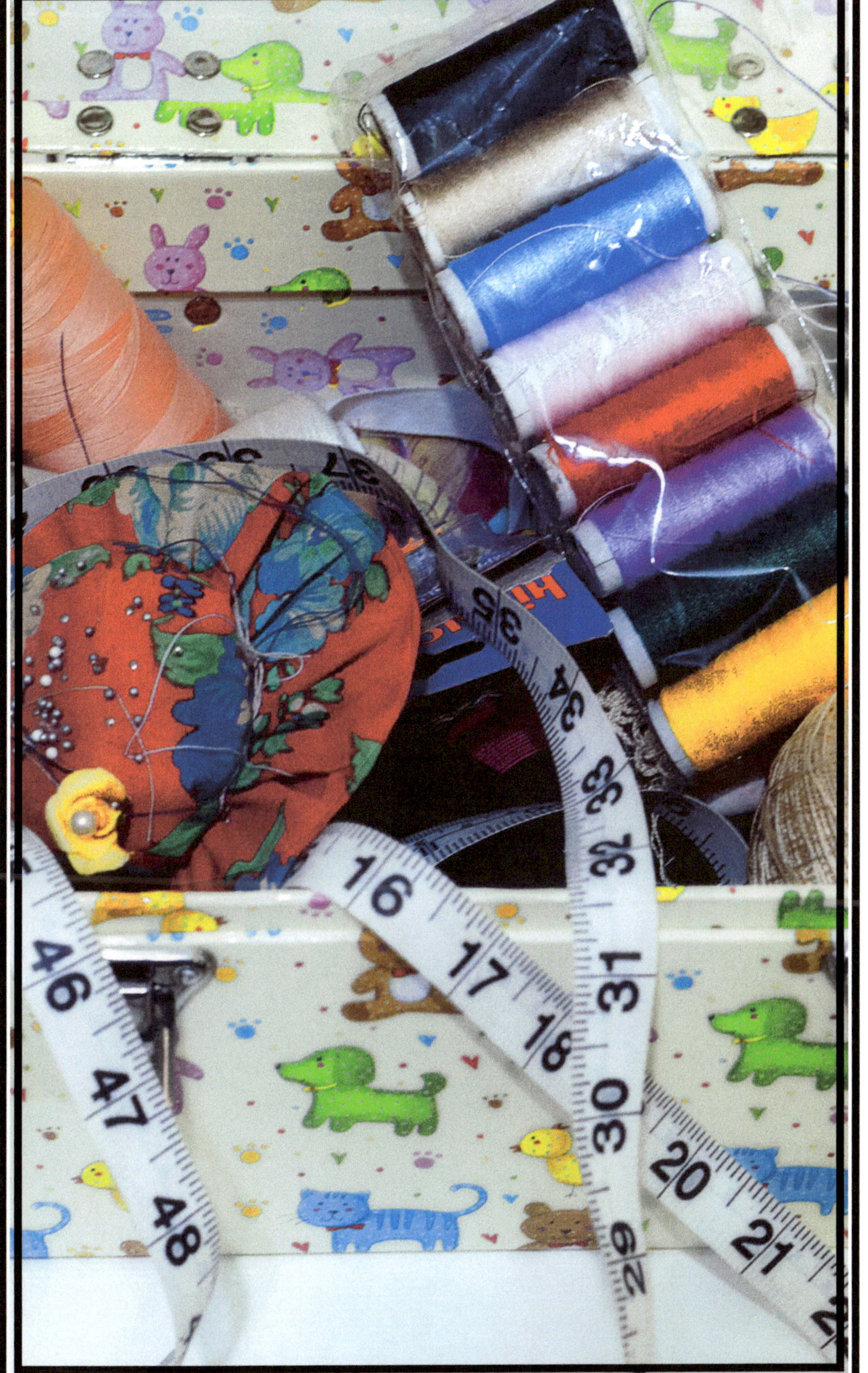

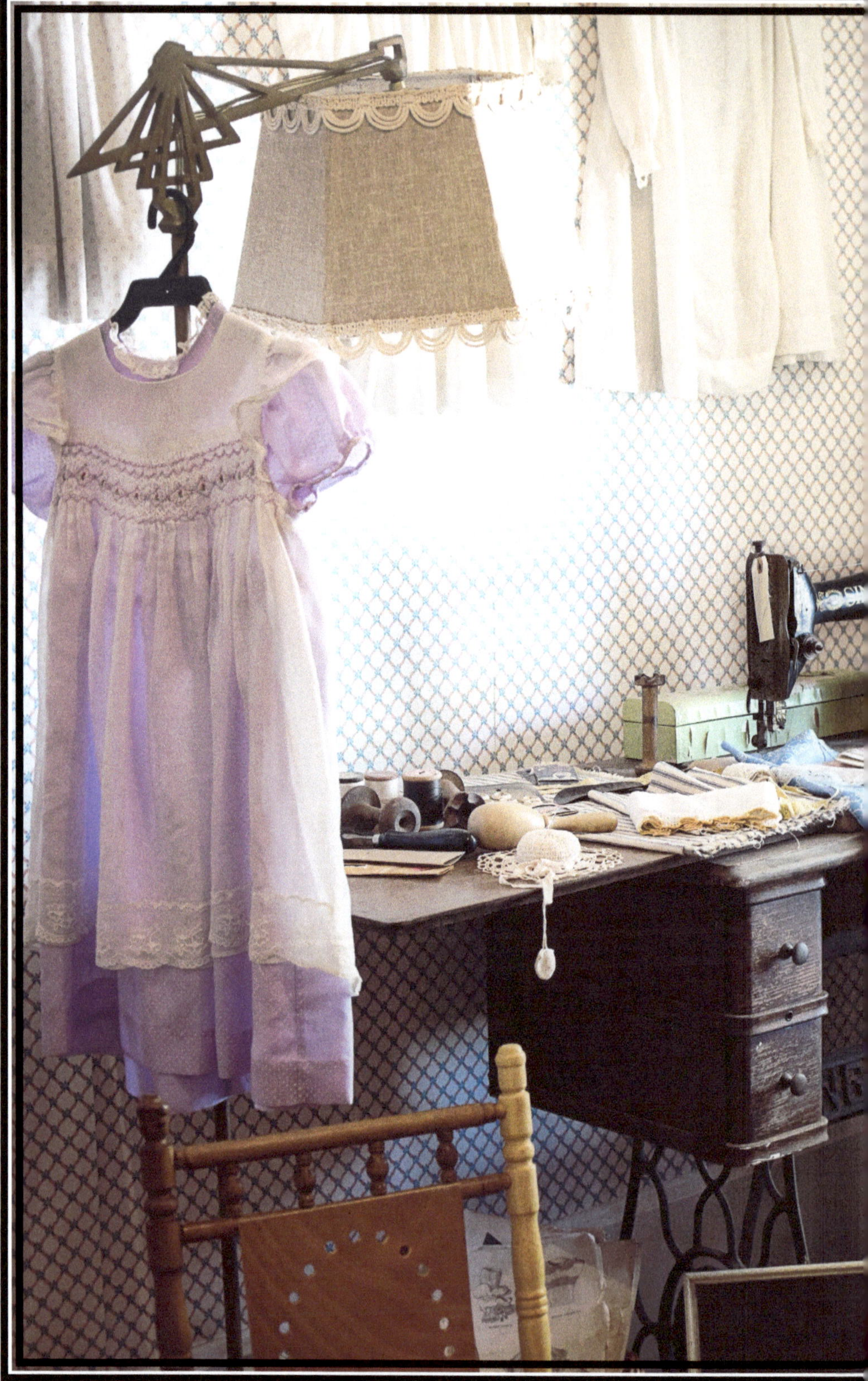

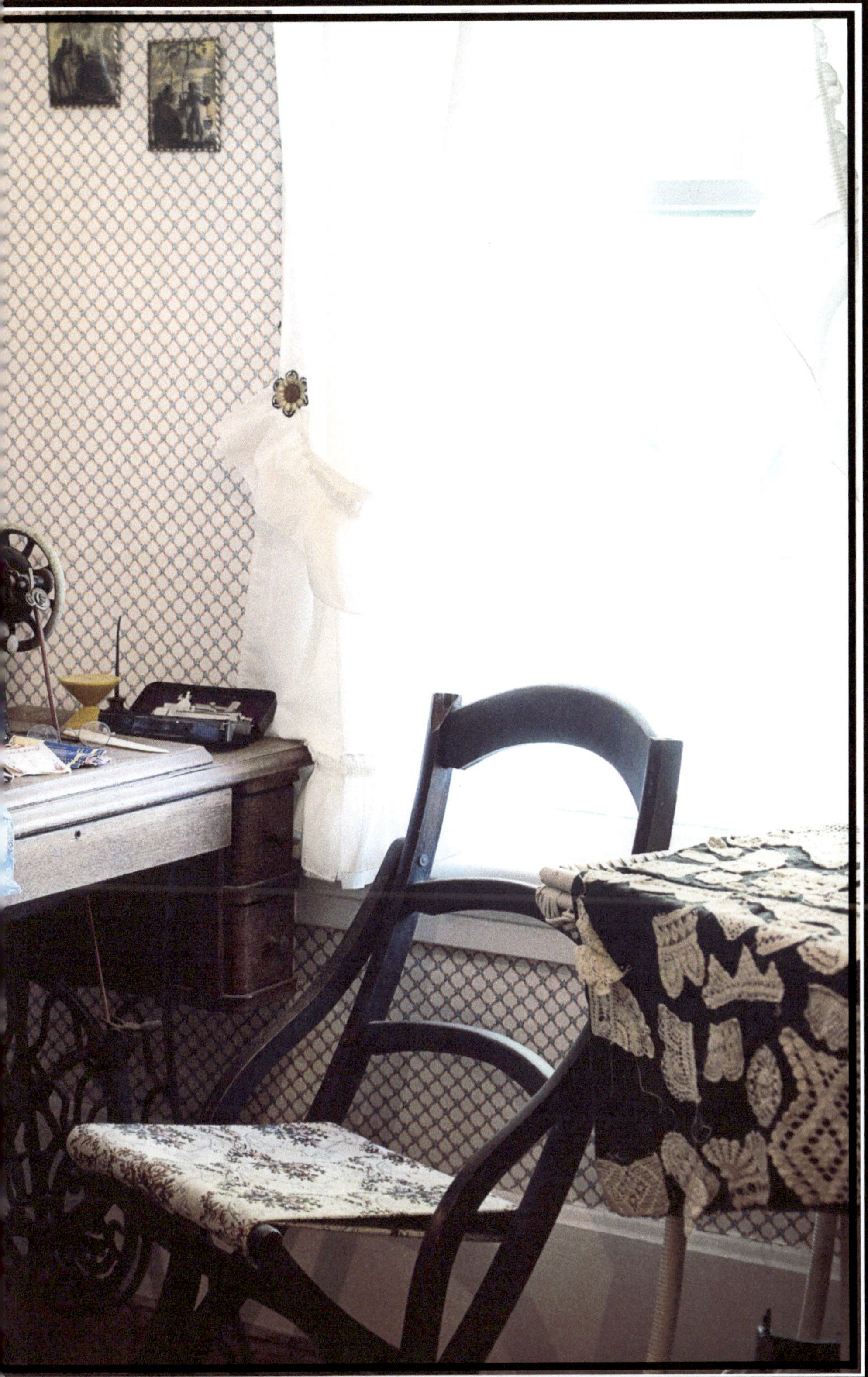

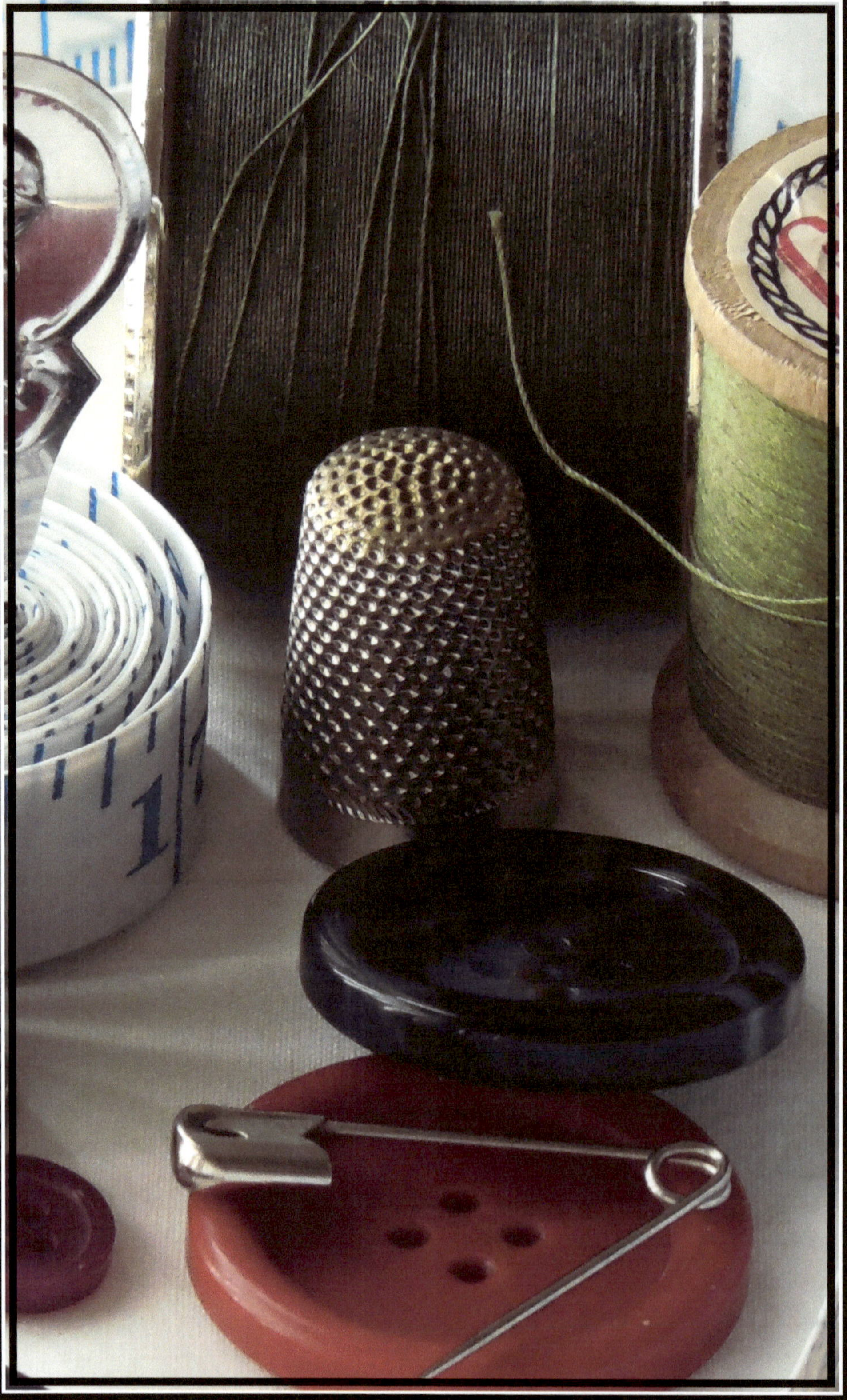

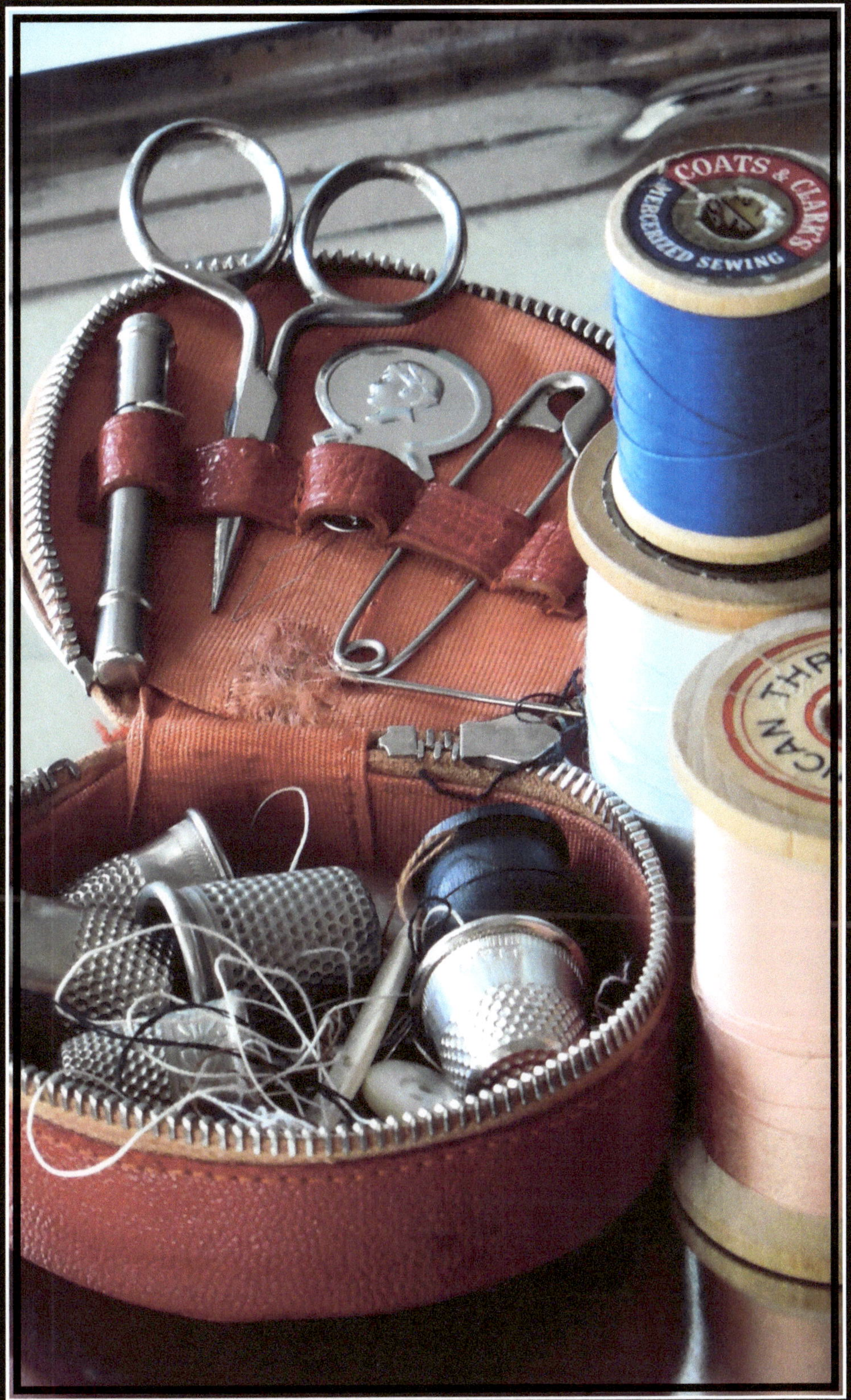
COATS & CLARK'S
MERCERIZED SEWING

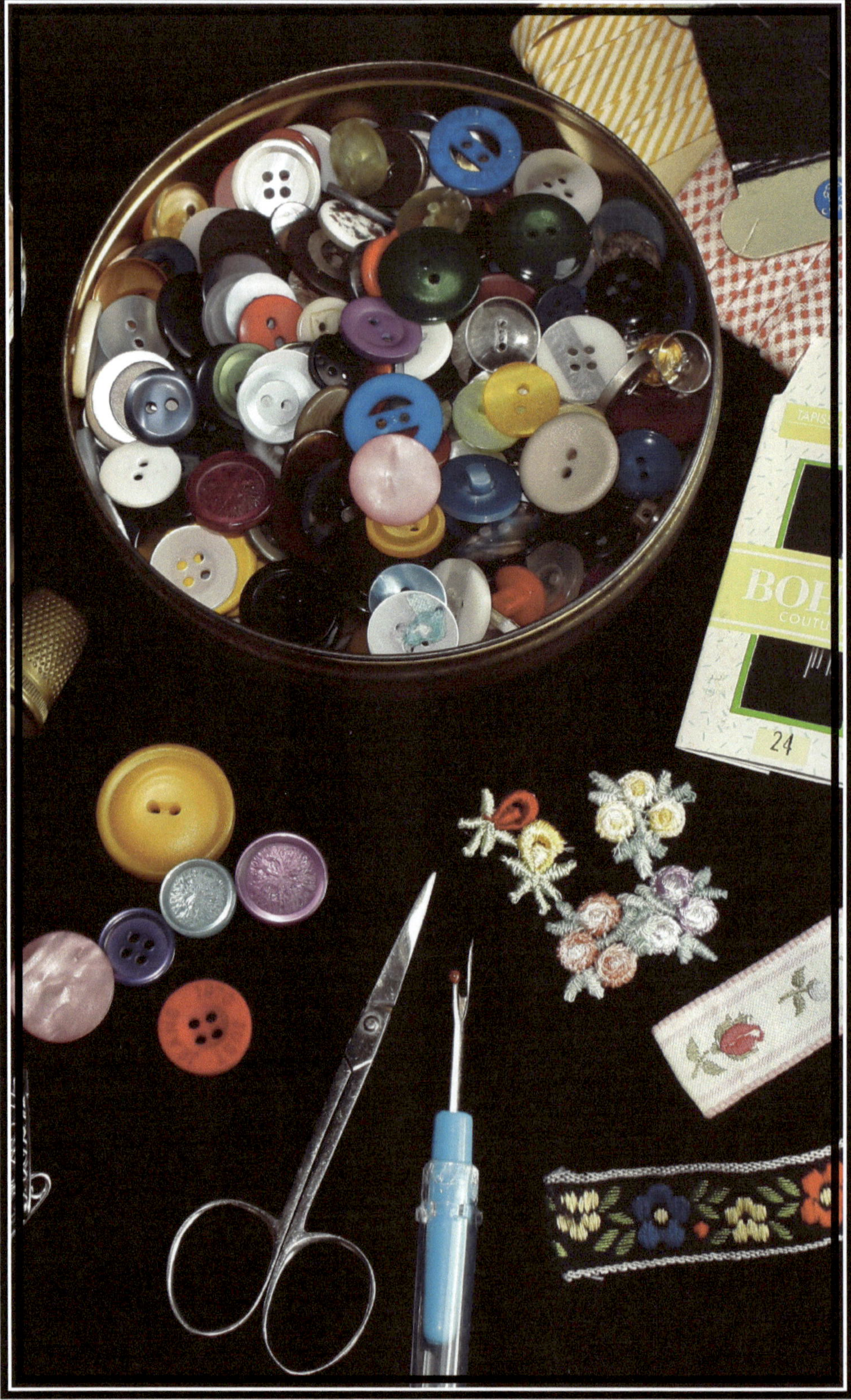

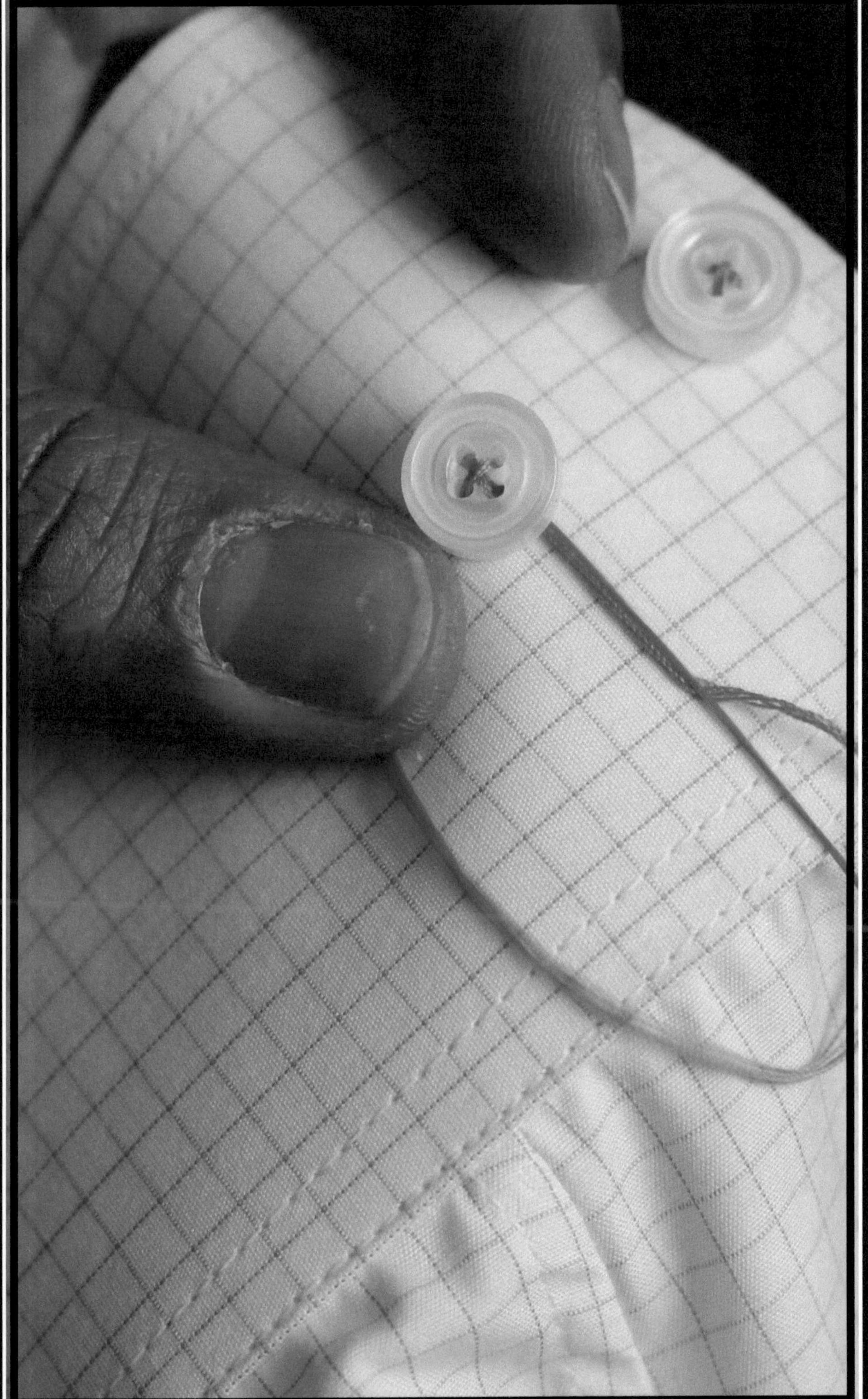

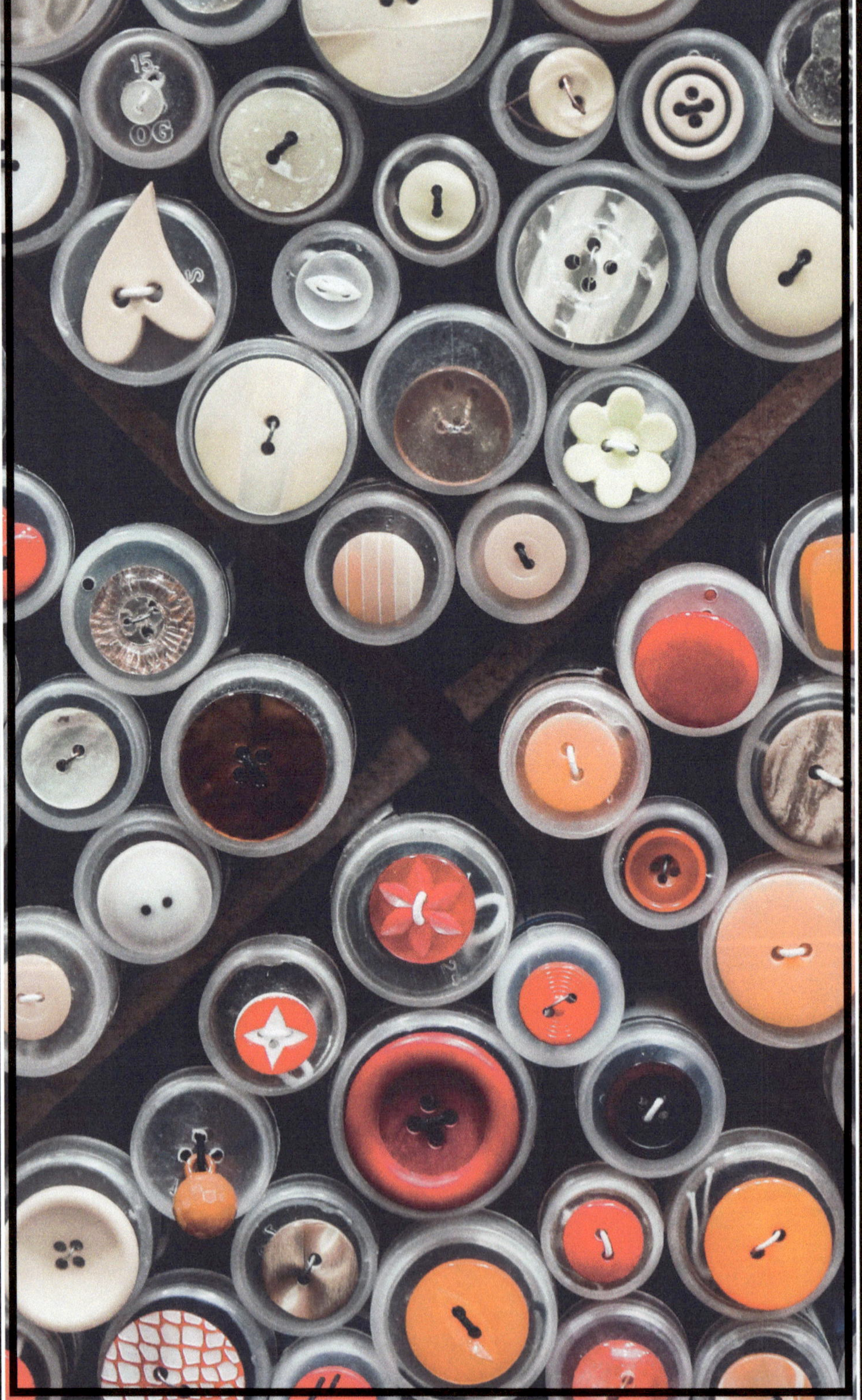

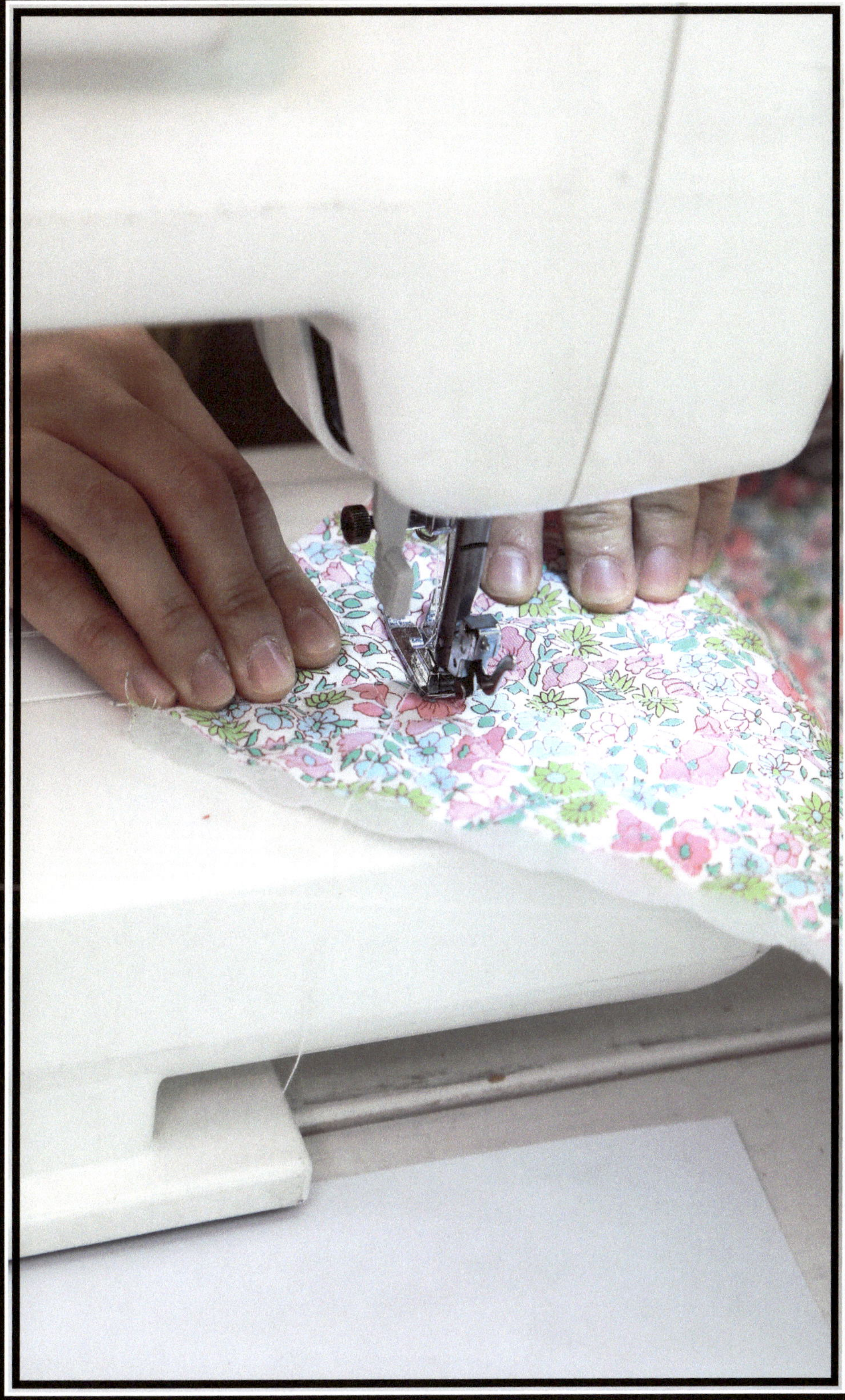

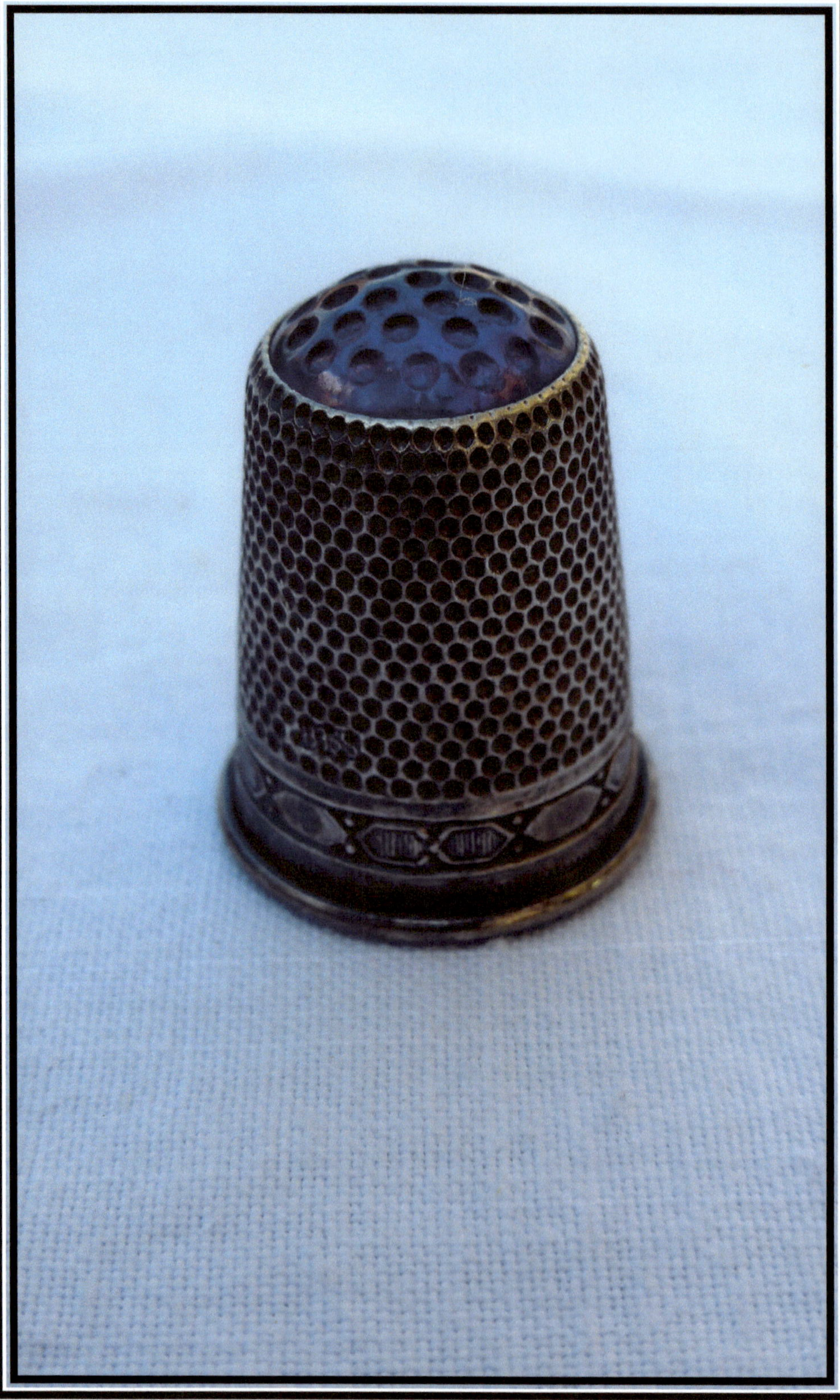

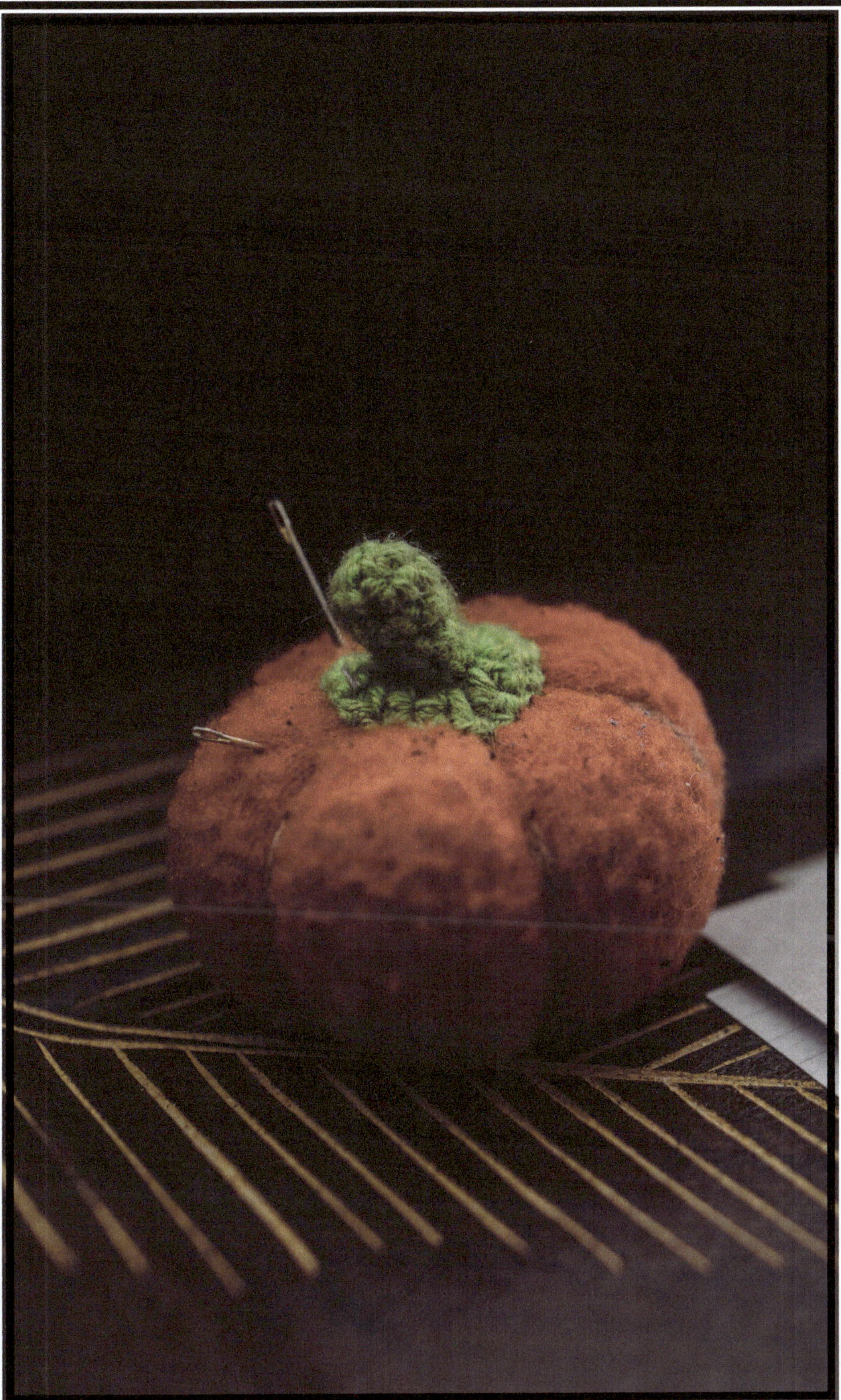

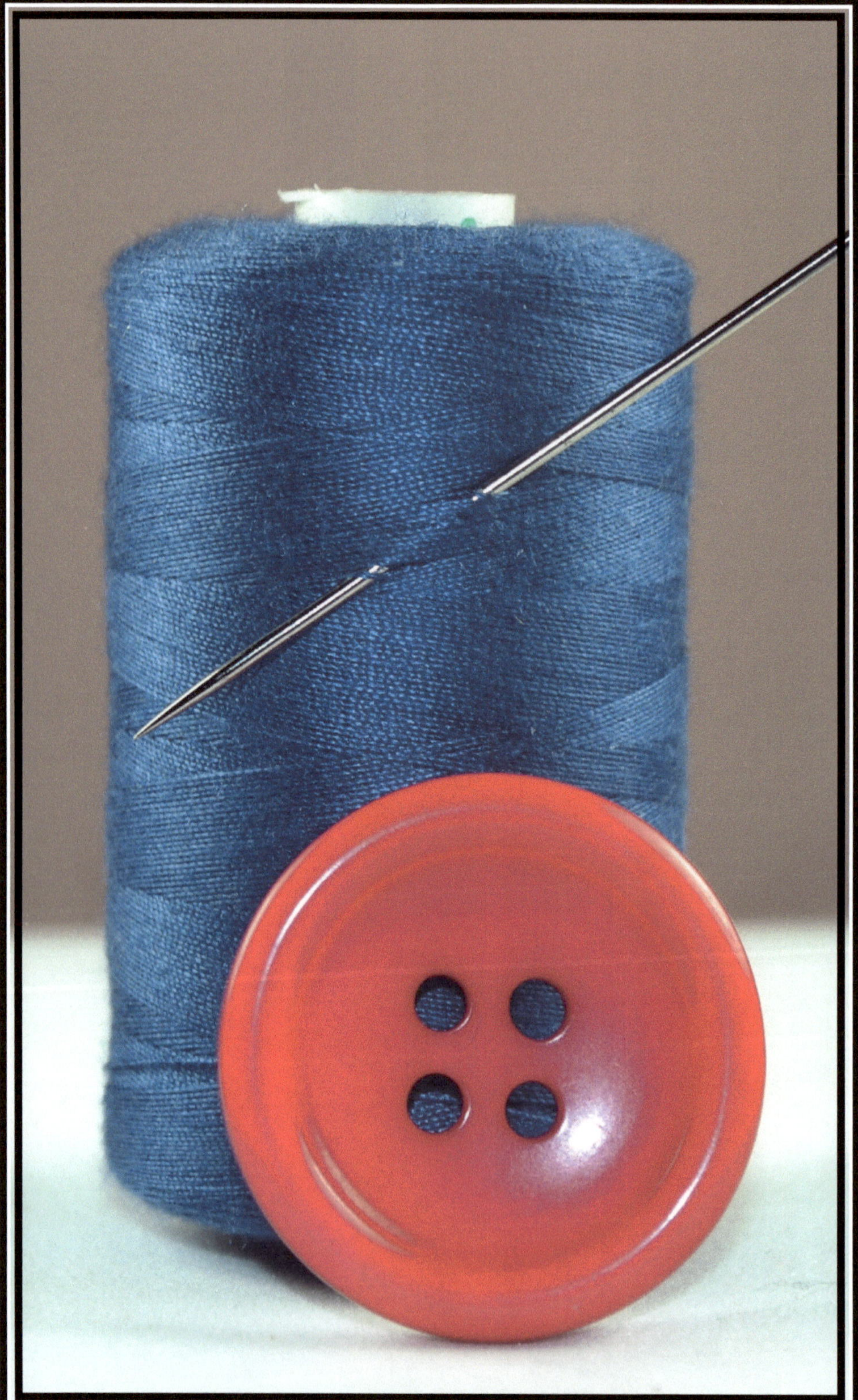

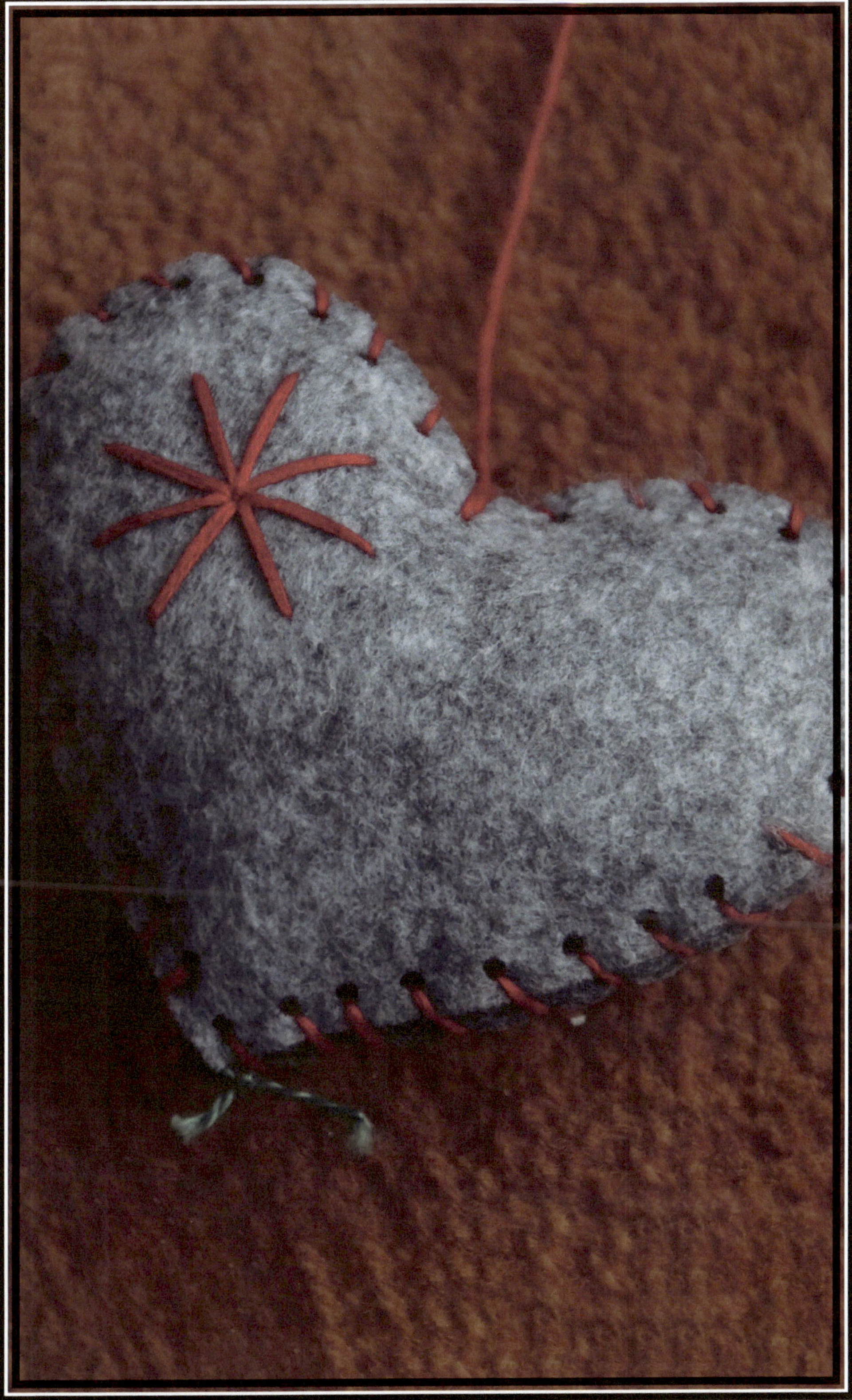

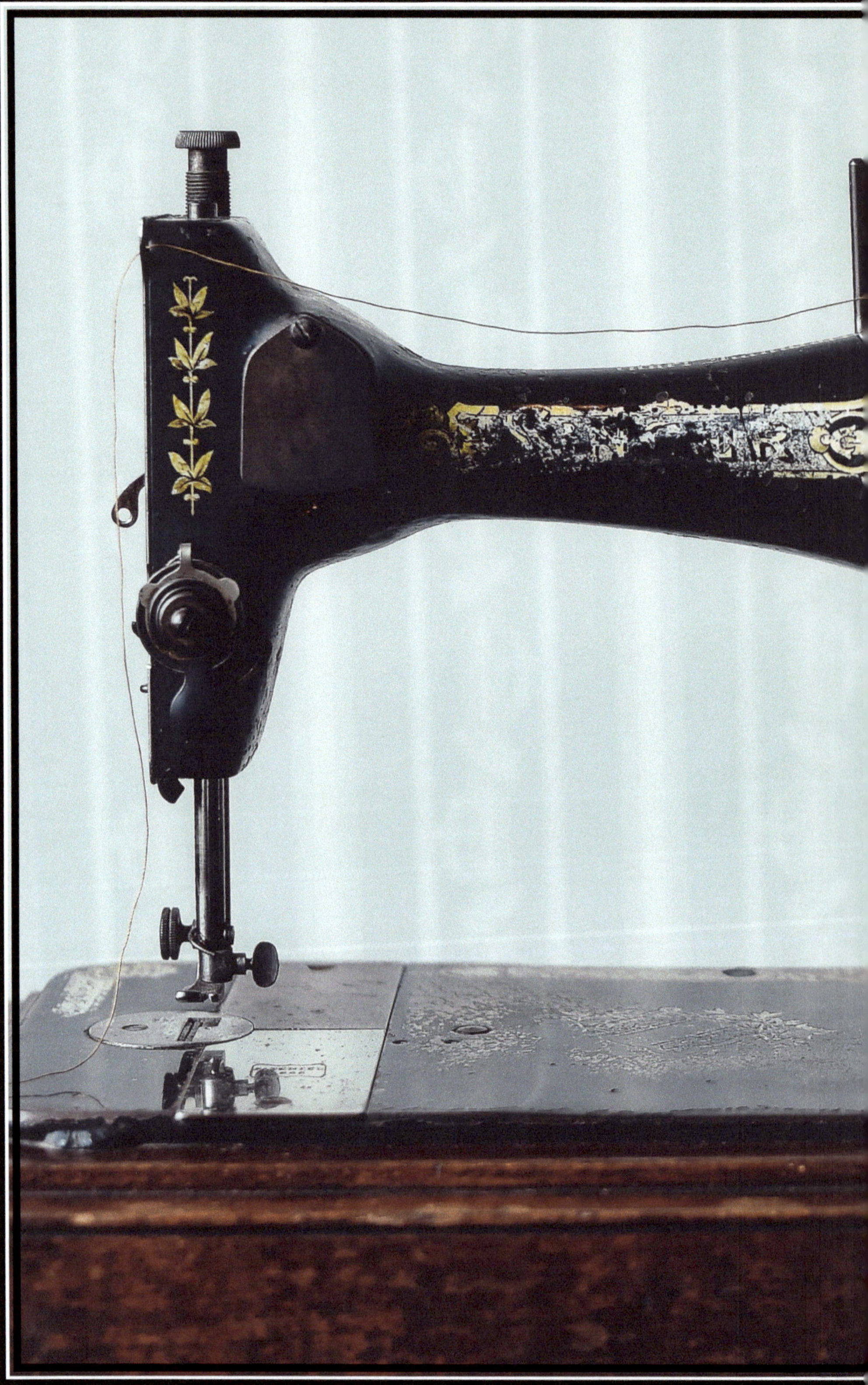

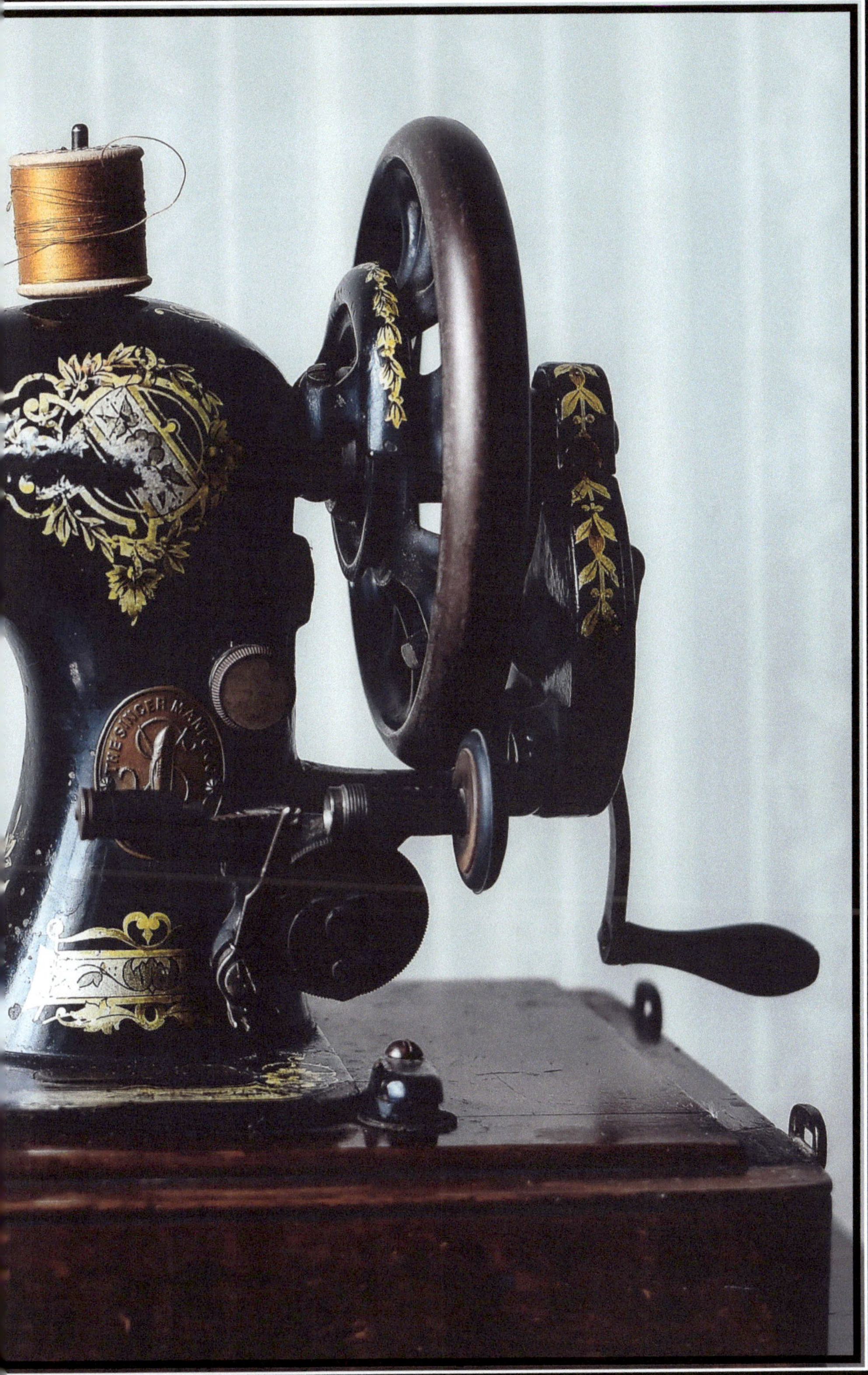

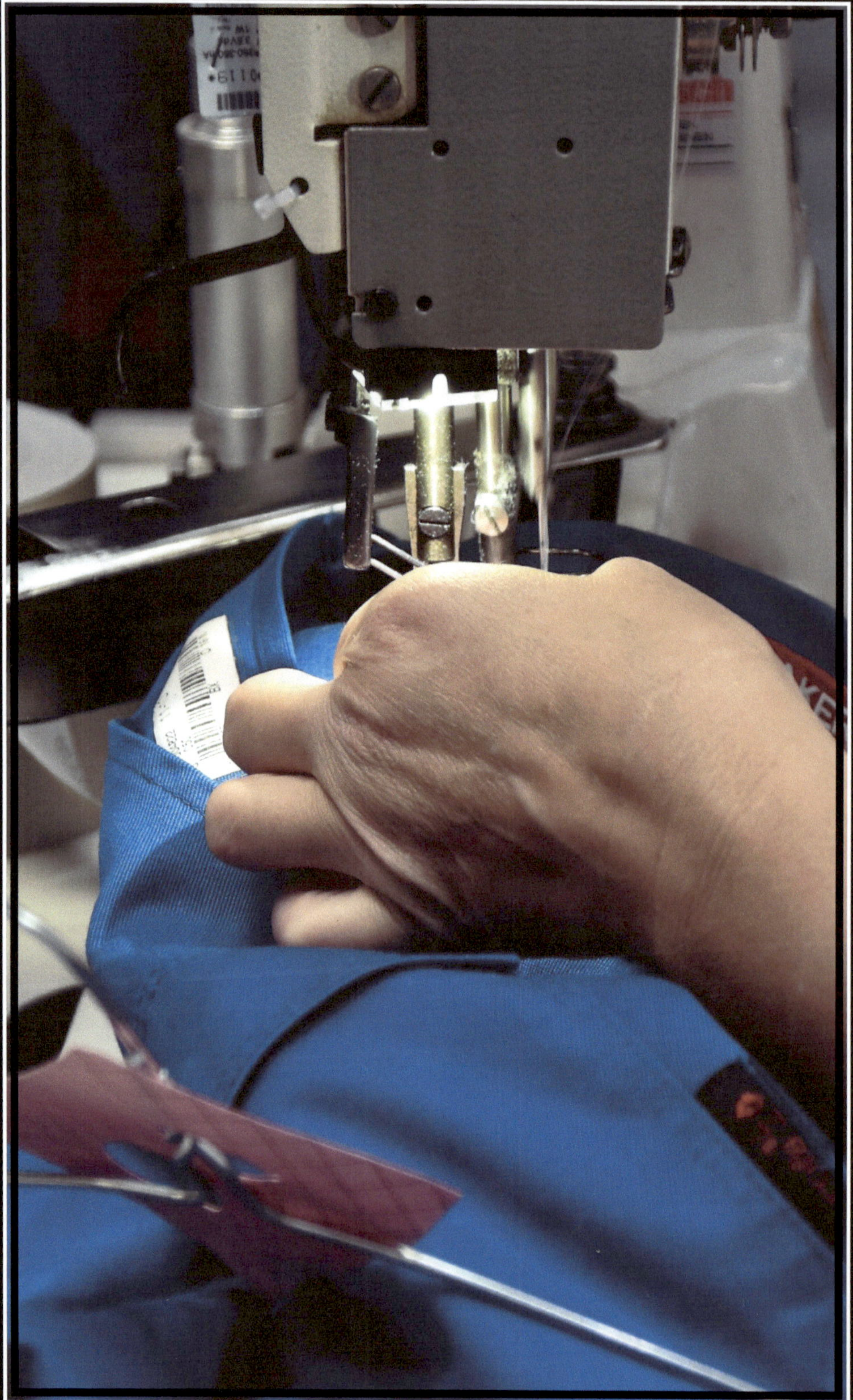

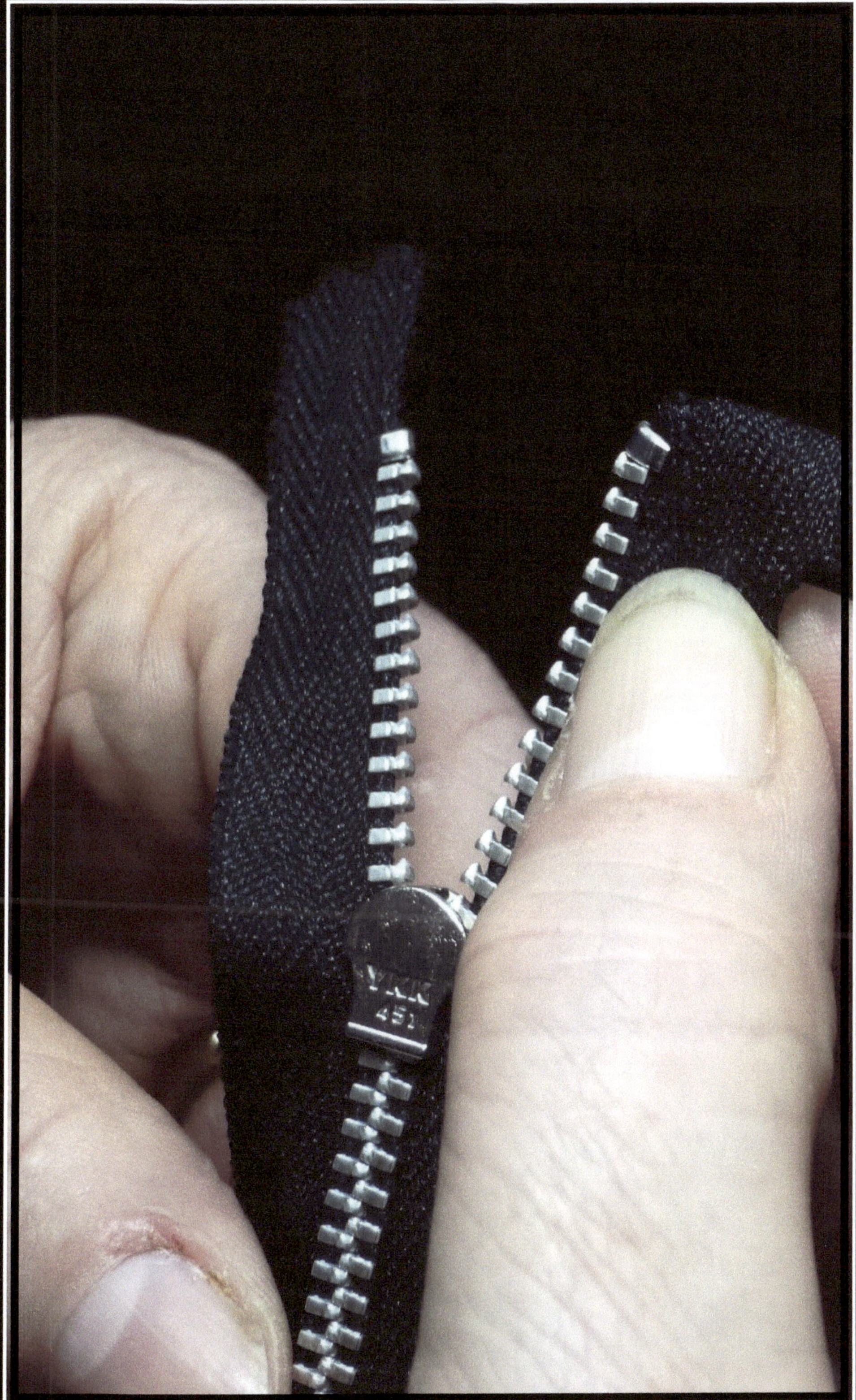